REWRITING THE SCRIPT:

A Doctor's Spiritual Journey Of Healing

JAMES WARPINSKI, MD

Rewriting the Script: A doctor's spiritual journey of healing

In the following discussions, all names of individuals are changed unless they have given explicit permission to use their real names.

The resources in this book are provided for informational purposes only and should not be used to replace the specialized training and professional judgment of a health care or mental health care professional.

Neither the author nor the publisher can be held responsible for the use of the information provided within this book. Please always consult a trained professional before making any decision regarding treatment of yourself or others.

ISBN: 979-8-9869094-0-0

This book is dedicated to my loving wife Diane who supported and encouraged me to be the husband and father God has called me to be.

The Lord is my light and my salvation; whom shall I fear?

Psalm 27:1 (NIV)

Table of Contents

Prologue:

Dad's Office

Children are a gift from the Lord.
They are a reward from him.
Happy is the man whose quiver is full of them!

Psalm 127:3,5a (NLT)

"Everybody get dressed in your Sunday clothes," Mom commanded. "We are all going to see Dad at his new office." Seeing Dad was always exciting for us kids. We didn't see him much anymore now that he had his own place to live. What was this all about? Would he be coming home?

Mom loaded us into the station wagon for the drive across town. I was old enough to claim one of the rear seats; a few of my younger siblings sat on the floor. I had been to Dad's other office many times before, and was surprised when we pulled into the parking lot of a small brick building in a strip mall next to a bakery and a dry cleaner. Dad's name was on the door. So, this was his new office? What happened to the other one, the new building he and his partners had built, brightly lit with lots of windows, a central courtyard and plenty of chairs in the waiting area? (I later learned he had left his old practice due to the social pressure of leaving his wife and kids. Fired? Forced out? We never talked about it.)

We piled out of the car and filled the small waiting room. There we sat, restlessly waiting for our turn to be called back to Dad's office, like any other family of patients on his busy schedule. Only we were the doctor's own family, ten puzzled children and their anxious mother.

Finally, the nurse ushered us back. My stomach churned as I joined the lineup in Dad's private office. Standing room only; there weren't enough chairs. Mom pressed Dad for an answer. "Are you really going to leave all of these children?" No verbal response, just a silent nod to the room full of confused children and their crying mother. I don't remember any words after that, only sick feelings and tears on the painful car ride home.

There's still some debate among my siblings and myself about the details of this event and if it even took place as I remember it. Who was there? What specific things were said? Could this be a false memory, constructed to make sense out of an incomprehensible situation? I don't know for sure, and I'm not sure it matters much now. The reality is, Dad left us to start a new life; Mom remained to raise us on her own.

Since that time, I've lived much of my life with a sense of being abandoned and left behind. I left home for that meeting as a member of a family with two parents. I returned with only one to be raised in a single parent household. The security I had known as a child left me behind that day as did my dad. I repeatedly asked myself, *Why was this happening? Were we kids somehow to blame? What will this mean for our family? Will we ever see dad again?* I didn't know that I'd spend most of my life trying to answer these questions and doing everything to keep from being abandoned like that ever again. And I resolved that I would never walk out on the people I loved.

For most of my life, this has been the story that defined me and shaped my approach to life, yet one too painful to share with others. My life changed forever that day. I was thirteen years old, and this was to be the point of no return for our family. Now, more than half a century later, I realize that telling my story may be the only way to overcome it.

PART ONE, EARLY LIFE:

FAITH IN THE BACKGROUND

Chapter 1

Origins

God determines the time and place where each one should live.

Acts 17:26 (NIV)

My earliest memory–reading to Dad

I was a young boy, newly learning to read, five or six years old. We lived in a one-story ranch with a finished basement, all fourteen of us. One evening, walking down the hall toward the main floor bathroom I spied my dad lying on his bed. Dressed only in large boxer shorts and a T-shirt, he was reading one of his ever-present medical books. On both nightstands alongside the bed lay piles of books, a small sample of the countless books and encyclopedias that filled up the living room, which doubled as our private library.

As I passed by the open bedroom door, Dad invited me to join him, and I readily accepted. This was a privilege rarely afforded children in our family: to be alone with Dad's full attention, and in his bedroom at that. We children never went into our parents' private sanctuary unless sent there on some mission by one of them. I don't actually recall ever being in that bedroom with Dad before or since. The bed was immense, many times the size of the single beds in our basement dormitory where I slept with three of my brothers. Dad was a large man, over 300 pounds, and climbing into bed next to him, I felt small but so secure. The words looked complicated, like nothing I had ever read before. I asked if I could read to him, and he said yes.

The massive book was too big for me to hold by myself, so he helped. I snuggled close and slowly sounded out the words one by one with his encouragement along the way. Together, we navigated the long and funny-sounding words in sentences that never seemed to come to an end. I didn't have any idea what the text meant, but there I was, nestled next to my dad in his bed, reading out of a book I could barely hoist.

I've thought a lot about that evening over the years, reading in bed with my dad. The image remains as sharp and clear as if it were just last night. But why does this particular incident stand preeminent in my storehouse of memories, coming alive day after day, year after year? What could it mean to me now? Could it be the overwhelming sense of acceptance and security, lying close to my dad, the one man big enough and strong enough to protect me from any harm? Maybe, but there's more to it than that. The glow of pride and accomplishment has never faded even over 60 years later. I would spend almost my entire life seeking Dad's approval, his encouragement and his love, just like that night. How much would I look to regain that through the substitutes I've recruited to take his place, second-stringers, never able to do the work of the starters? How often would I try to impress people when I learned something or gained some new ability? Does this all trace back to that evening in bed reading to my dad?

I grew up in a wonderful family at a time when family, neighborhood, and church were seamlessly interconnected. Ours was a traditional 1950s' Norman Rockwell home in a typical neighborhood in a White working-class American city. The neighbors came from different walks of life: an engineer, a laborer, office worker, gas station owner, seamstress, and many others, raising a generation of baby boomers. Ours was the only doctor's family many of them knew. We all belonged to the same parish, and the children attended St. Philip's Catholic School. The men went off to work each morning and the women stayed home to keep house and raise their families while keeping an eye on each other's kids. As children, we felt safe, surrounded by a loving family and caring neighbors.

Within a few blocks of home, we had a couple of small grocery stores, two restaurants, and a drive-in theater. Kids played in the city park at the end of the street where a supervised park shelter provided recreation and daytime childcare throughout the summer months. Adults came to the park at night to play softball under the lights. Next to the park, lay a small swamp for boys to explore and build their secret hideouts. The East River marked the boundary of the park, offered fishing and boating in the summer, and dared the adventurous to walk on the ice in the winter.

Meet my family

My parents were both descendants of self-reliant nineteenth-century immigrants. Dad's grandfather came from Poland to Chicago. Some held that these Polish forebears were fugitive horse thieves, which made for rather exciting stories. The truth is more likely that my great-grandfather and his brother came to America to avoid being conscripted into Kaiser Wilhelm's army. Years later, my grandfather and his brother moved to the Green Bay area to live in the town of Poland, Wisconsin.

Mom's grandmother traveled to America smuggled in a box! She and three men from a village in Bohemia were on their way to the Bremen seaport when a purse snatcher stole her handbag with her ticket. She had worked and saved for a year to buy that ticket. Now what was she to do? One of her fellow immigrants was a carpenter who had built a steamer chest for the passage, just the right size for their diminutive companion. Onto the ship for America they went, the three men and my great grandma, the stowaway.

Everyone we knew considered Dad to be the brightest person they had ever met. He learned to read early on, skipped a couple of grades in school, and entered medical school at 20, married my mom three months later. They had their first child within a year and the second 18 months after that. Dad still graduated second in his class. While Dad got all the attention for his intelligence and accomplishment as a doctor, Mom became the one who had the greatest impact on my education, from ensuring that homework was done to ferrying me to after school programs (and meeting with the principal on more than one occasion). She had left school after eighth grade to help at home and eventually fulfilled her lifelong dream to graduate from high school by earning her High School Equivalency degree at age sixty-five.

This is the family I was born into–hardworking, independent, determined to make a new and better life for themselves and their children. In a sense, they embodied the post-World War II American dream. Like many descendants of immigrants, my siblings and I had no exposure to the home country apart from tasting some special foods and catching occasional bits of our ancestors' native languages chiefly when our parents had something they didn't want us to understand. At these times, they spoke to each other in a mixture of Polish and Bohemian, a cryptic code we kids were never able to break. Otherwise, it was English all the time.

South Dakota living

Although our parents grew up on farms near Green Bay, we always thought of ourselves as being well-traveled. Most people born in the area never left except for a few who had visited places like Mount Rushmore. We had actually lived in South Dakota for a time, and I was even born there. Other than that, my parents had never lived far away from their families except for medical school in Milwaukee, internship 30 miles from home followed by a rural practice a full 60 miles away.

But Dad dreamed of bigger things. He wanted to serve the Native American people. The family, now numbering four children, moved west to the small town of McLaughlin in north central South Dakota next to the Standing Rock Indian Reservation. This was the country of Sitting Bull and the Sioux Indians. The community agreed to open a hospital and clinic if doctors would come there to practice.

Those were exciting days for our family, ones still recalled with a sort of mystical fondness, the days when our parents were unmistakably in love and added four children in five years. There were rodeos, fairs, and small-town life and wide-open spaces where one man reportedly owned an entire county. There was the story of Sitting Bull secretly buried in a concrete grave overlooking the Missouri River. There were long but exciting car rides back to Wisconsin in the days before the Interstate Highway, fast food, and disposable diapers. Mom told of stopping at gas stations along the way to rinse out the cloth diapers, then hanging them out the car windows to dry, flapping in the wind at fifty-five miles per hour. And there were a lot of diapers.

The story of our time in McLaughlin was one of the doctor and his growing family assuming a prominent position in the community. Coming to serve in a rural area meant great sacrifice. Physicians now practice at a time when medicine is increasingly treated as a business. The doctor-patient relationship is seen as a transaction brokered by the insurance company. But not in those days when doctors were sought after and respected, and a patient might bring in a couple of chickens or some eggs to settle their account.

I don't have many firsthand memories of our time in South Dakota, though it has been reported that I once planted a money tree in our yard. On another occasion, I was canvassing the neighborhood one stormy afternoon looking for cookies when a tornado blew through our small town. One of our neighbors took me inside to ride out the storm but there was no way for them to get in touch with my family. My anxious parents spent the storm wondering whatever could have happened to little Jimmy.

In spite of the demands on Dad's time, life in McLaughlin was good for our family until tragedy struck. Susie was the third oldest child in our family. As a toddler, she developed rheumatic fever, a complication of a strep throat. In fighting off the strep infection, the body's immune system attacks the heart and destroys the heart valves. Susie was desperately ill and required all of Mom's attention since our extended family lived over twelve hours away. Despite repeated trips to the Mayo Clinic, Susie eventually died at the age of six from heart failure. Penicillin had only recently been discovered, too late to prevent her death. Within several months, our family moved back to Wisconsin to be closer to home; the South Dakota adventure had come to an end. None of us knew it at the time, but events occurring in South Dakota would leave their mark on our family far beyond the fond memories.

Our family never talked about that hasty return from South Dakota, about the heartache and pain of losing a child while living 700 miles from home. We never discussed the pressure Mom must have felt as our family kept growing while Dad was busy in the hospital and clinic in the day and then taking care of emergencies and house calls at night. Years later, I would come to realize that these same unspoken questions and challenges would apply to my own life as a husband, father, and doctor. I could only wonder how knowing their answers might have affected my own life.

Chapter 2

Life on Louise St.

Train up a child in the way he should go;
even when he is old he will not depart from it.

Proverbs 22:6 (ESV)

Crowded but happy

Both of my parents had grown up on farms where the children worked every day to make their contribution to the family. That expectation carried over to me and my siblings with our regular chores around the house and jobs in the neighborhood. Early mornings in late June, we rode our bikes to a nearby farm to pick strawberries, an ideal summer job for pre-teens. Like the Biblical laborers in the vineyard, we waited to be chosen to pick in a designated area of the field. At the going rate of seven cents per quart, a good week of picking might net the diligent laborer several dollars, a small fortune in those days. The picking was supervised by a strict crew who ensured that we didn't overlook any strawberries and didn't eat any either. For quality assurance, we needed to ensure that the strawberries were ripe and ready for consumption. Unfortunately, the overseers didn't agree with our commitment to excellence, nor did they look kindly on the strawberry fights we would occasionally have out in the field. Ideally, when the supervisor was looking the other way, one of us would try to hit one of the others in the mid-back with a particularly juicy strawberry. Mom didn't care much for this entertainment either when laundry time came.

Ours was a traditional Catholic family in which both my parents were named after Mary, the mother of Jesus. Marion and Marian, same name, different spellings. Catholic families in those days were often large with five, six, or seven children; eight or more was nothing unusual. One of my parents' friends even had eighteen children.

It seemed like my mother was always pregnant, giving birth to fourteen children over a span of seventeen years with no twins. Our family was a group of individual cohorts. Mary Barbara and Kathy, the older sisters, ever in command, were followed by Susie. Next came "the Four Boys," Mark, Joe, Jim, and John. Coming up next were the five girls, Margaret, Jane, Nancy, Amy, and Lora. Bringing up the rear were Luke and Lucy. This made me number six in the sequence, in the middle third of the family. I once read about the way birth order affects one's life prospects and outcomes. How would this apply to a family like ours? Each of the cohorts seemed to have its own "oldest" and "youngest" member. However I looked at it, I was always in the middle where loyalty, compromise, and peace-keeping prevail.

Unless you were there, it may be hard to imagine all these people, Mom, Dad, and thirteen children in a three-bedroom, two-bath, single-story family home with overflow accommodations in the partially finished basement. To anyone else, it probably looked like any other ordinary house. For me, every room was special in its own way, each representing the idealized life of a young boy growing up into the American dream of the 1950s.

Entering the front door, we were greeted by a large picture of Jesus and his parents, the Holy Family, the ideal for our home. Ahead, the kitchen formed the center of the home in so many ways. Down the hallway to the left were the three official bedrooms and the coveted upstairs bathroom where one of my sisters used to hide books between the windows.

Most families eat their meals at a table in the kitchen or dining room. Not us, especially for breakfast. There wasn't enough room for all of us to eat in the kitchen. The younger children ate at the snack bar, the youngest in the ever-present highchair. The next oldest were relegated to eat sitting on the kitchen floor up against the cabinets or back door. Late arrivals ate their meals on the basement steps. On special occasions, we ate at the dining room table. Dad was usually gone for work before we had breakfast, and he wasn't often home for dinner either. When he had a particularly busy day at work, the kids would be sent off to the nearby cafe or pizza parlor for dinner while our parents enjoyed a few minutes of peace and quiet.

The kitchen also housed the lunch assembly production line. One of the kids would lay out all the slices from two loaves of bread, dealing them out like cards at a casino. Another was assigned the responsibility for spreading Miracle Whip on alternate slices. This required a great degree of skill to keep from making a mess of the whole area. The third production worker applied a slice of bologna or salami and an occasional slice of processed cheese. Next, each sandwich unit was wrapped in waxed paper, and the production supervisor checked to make sure we had enough for everyone. On special occasions, ham salad (affectionately known as "party meat") replaced the bologna. Fridays were meatless as ordered by the Catholic Church, so we would see either peanut butter or cheese, typically smothered in Welch's grape jelly.

The usual school lunch contained two sandwiches for the older kids and one for each of the younger ones, a couple of store-bought cookies, and an apple (oranges and bananas were rare treats). The final step involved assembling our rations into paper lunch bags and lining them up on the kitchen counter where they stood overnight at attention awaiting morning reveille.

Mom didn't cook a lot of fancy meals; her signature dish was ring bologna with mashed potatoes and cream style corn. Fridays, especially in Lent, meant Campbell's tomato soup and grilled cheese sandwiches. Otherwise, Aunt Anna or one of Mom's household helpers prepared most of our meals. Once, Mom planned to make a cherry dessert, but she couldn't locate the canned pie filling. It had mysteriously vanished from our kitchen. A search and rescue effort ensued, and the empty can was located under the basement steps where Joe and I had hidden the evidence.

The living room served as our private chapel where Mom assembled us for evening prayers and the rosary, each of us kneeling before the crucifix hanging over the fireplace mantle. On either side of the fireplace, Dad's private reference library filled the bookcases from floor to ceiling with complete sets of up-to-date encyclopedias: *World Book*, *Encyclopedia Britannica,* as well as several science encyclopedias. A leather-bound set of *Great Books* beckoned any reader brave enough to give them a try. We all professed to cherish these books above all the others, though we mostly resisted their siren call. Most revered of all the books was the oversized family Bible with its dates of all the important family events: marriages, births, and deaths. If the county library ever ran short of books, our home was on standby.

Reading was a feature of our family life for as long as I could remember. Dad's reading set an example for the whole family. As a child, he would often hide from his cousins and playmates in a ditch or a culvert with a book in hand. I shared Dad's love for encyclopedias and dictionaries but without a culvert handy, I would shoehorn myself into a spot on the living room floor between the couch and bookcase where I often read articles and looked up words or subjects for the sheer enjoyment of learning, hoping to avoid getting stepped on by one of the younger kids.

The kids mostly slept in the two downstairs bedrooms, each with a small window through which a child or teen could squeeze in an emergency or at other times. The four boys slept in their barracks; my younger sisters occupied the other bedroom, the one where the sleeping girls were often awakened by strange noises. Margaret slept in a closet in "the girls' room."

A bathroom, laundry room, furnace room and workroom for Dad's electronics gear completed the basement. Luke, my youngest brother, slept in the furnace room under the duct work, with a thoughtful reminder to brush his teeth written on the ceiling, courtesy of one of my sisters. With access to Dad's electronics gear, Luke wired speakers in the ceiling and behind a poster in the girls' room to issue morning wake-up calls and other annoying sounds.

I didn't have to worry about all the noise in such a crowded setting, as I grew up deaf in my right ear, the permanent result of measles. I remember seeing the Ear, Nose and Throat specialist who gave my parents and me the bad news: I would never be able to hear out of my right ear. In a way, being deaf in one ear worked to my advantage, as I could sleep on my left side in blissful silence.

The boys and girls in our family did share one thing every school morning, the intense competition for the downstairs bathroom. Four boys, six girls, one cramped bathroom. Woe to the boy who missed his chance before the girls got started. I needed to get in line early to beat the rush, especially if I wanted to enjoy the limited supply of hot water.

Nocturnal adventures

Once the household quieted down for the day, the kids were sent to bed for the night, but it would be common for one or more to squeeze through a bedroom window to explore the neighborhood in the dark. Not that there was anywhere to go. Sometimes, we would head off to the store to buy candy or soda. Other times, it would be rewarding enough to know that we managed to escape the house undetected, like prisoners eluding their guards.

The high point of these nighttime breakouts would be to station ourselves behind the nearby Starlight Drive-in Theater. We couldn't exactly make out what the actors on screen were saying, but that didn't matter to us. Many of the cars had the window speakers turned up, so we could sort of hear the dialogue. Better yet, sometimes, the movies were rated for older teens and adults, a forbidden temptation for young boys. Regardless of the movie, the thought of being outside in the cool summer evening weather was delightful in its own way. Knowing that we weren't supposed to be there made it that much more attractive.

We weren't exactly a family of backpackers. Getting out in nature meant sleeping in a large canvas army surplus tent with its unmistakable musty smell, like sleeping in an old tennis shoe. Situated under a hickory tree, the tent served as headquarters of our camping expeditions. We slept on our mattresses which we dragged up the stairs from our bedroom. In true suburban roughing-it fashion, we ran an extension cord out the backdoor and across the backyard to the tent. Our campsite was now complete with lights, mattresses, pillows, blankets and an ample supply of food.

Camping in the backyard was something only the older kids got to do. One night, Mark and Joe invited me to join them and some of the older neighborhood boys. I was even invited to participate in their favorite pastime, trading baseball cards! Each boy would bring his personal collection to these evening exchanges hoping to find a coveted card. Usually, we would buy these cards at DeLeers grocery store a few blocks away from our house. Each pack of cards came with a thin piece of gum and trading cards bearing players' pictures and statistics. Best of all, each came with the hope that it contained a prized rookie card of one of the Milwaukee Braves, our favorite team. With his stack of cards in hand, each boy would lay out some of his favorites and see if he could trade for a more favorable specimen. Trading sessions usually went well except for one night when the campout had a special guest.

Wayne, also known as "Beaver," was the oldest and strongest boy in the neighborhood (he could hit a home run left-handed). One summer night, he joined us in the tent with his impressive collection of baseball cards. Let the trading begin! Shortly after we started, a toxic fume filled the tent. Mass evacuation ensued as we gasped for fresh air and escaped with our lives. If only Dad had gotten gas masks at the army surplus store. In our rush to safety, we left all our prized baseball cards behind. When the air cleared, we returned to the tent only to find that some of our most prized cards had gone missing. Suspiciously, Beaver had remained in the tent, seemingly immune to the poisonous fumes. None of us had the courage to confront him about the missing cards or his unauthorized use of gas warfare.

Other times in the backyard, the campers would sneak off to DeLeers to pick up more provisions for our outdoor adventures. We were under strict orders not to leave the yard at night. In retrospect, that prohibition was all the inducement we needed to sneak away. I never actually got into trouble doing anything during these night time excursions, but I suspect a few of my sisters might have snuck out of their basement window with other things in mind besides watching a drive-in movie or trading baseball cards.

Neighborhood

Apart from camping during the summer, we didn't spend much time in the backyard, preferring the excitement and freedom of the park, an endless source of activity and adventure. Each morning, Mom sent us older kids out the door after breakfast forbidding us to return home until lunch time. Even the backyard was off limits during the day. Mom knew we would be safe and well-occupied at the park at the end of our block, and she could take care of the little kids at home. Fortunately, being banished from our own backyard never seemed like much of an inconvenience.

Bordered on three sides by a river and swamp, the park not only offered us secret hideouts and forts but also made it possible for us to recruit subjects for our scientific studies. This was the time when space exploration was becoming a national preoccupation. At the park, my fellow explorers and I deployed water rockets to send small amphibian astronauts (typically frogs or toads) into space. Upon their reentry, we would examine them for any ill effects of their atmospheric travels. In general, the dazed frogs usually hopped away after their interstellar adventure. In modern times, they would have entered a concussion protocol.

At the park, we also enjoyed playing baseball and board games like chess, all organized by the college-aged parkies. We went fishing for carp in the East River, though no one ever ate them. Summers meant clean, wholesome fun. That is, except for the enterprising neighbor kid with a unique business plan. He prided himself by finding dead frogs, which he baked on a hot tin roof before affixing them to pieces of cardboard to be sold as souvenirs of the park experience.

In the neighborhood, my friend, Gary, and I started our own club. Membership was restricted to boys in our grade living on our side of the street. This was a rather exclusive group. The club's rigid entrance requirements prevented my younger brother and the boy across the street from becoming members. Since a respectable club needs a club house or meeting place, Gary and I nailed a small placard bearing the name of the club and its two members in a tree in his front yard. We would occasionally climb up the tree to admire our exalted status as the founding and only members of our club.

Gary and I also enjoyed collecting coins, always on the alert for the coveted 1909S VDB Lincoln penny and the 1950 D Jefferson nickel. I had obtained one of those prized nickels and took it to a coin shop to be examined, but it had dropped onto the floor and rolled into a crack. The owner said he never found the nickel, much to my lasting dismay. About forty years later, I received a card with a 1950 D nickel from Gary. A true friend!

Early work

How can a young boy support his habit of soda, candy, and baseball cards? Aside from mowing lawns, the next best option in our household was babysitting, from which I learned a lot about being responsible for the welfare of young children. The income from babysitting was good but dependent on the law of supply and demand, and there was a large supply of babysitters in our household. I needed something more predictable than finding a rare coin that could be sold for a profit.

Early one December, I made the first major purchase of my life, a paper route, for $100 which was more money than I had ever seen. In those days, a paper route with its sixty to seventy-five customers was a coveted business opportunity, as reflected by the price. It was thrilling to pay back the full amount within the first couple of months thanks to the Christmas tips. I attributed the generosity of the customers to my attentive customer service. Without a bicycle of my own, I usually delivered papers on foot and became pretty adept at tossing papers onto the front porch while power walking on the sidewalk. Only rarely did a paper ever land on the roof, but many times, I had to dig through the bushes to retrieve an errant projectile.

Owning and operating a paper route also taught me a lot about financial management and how to make sacrifices when needed to keep my paper route going. My route started over one mile from home where I picked up my papers and delivered them in that neighborhood. My brother Mark had an adjacent paper route so we often worked together, especially on Sundays. Starting early, we could attend Mass, deliver our papers, head down to Kaap's for a sweet roll, and then spend the rest of the day golfing.

We walked the route in the winter; there was no way that my mother could have given us a ride to deliver papers. Who would have watched all the kids at home? In addition to providing needed spending money, the paper route helped me start saving for college using the popular "Christmas Club" program designed for young savers. Each week, we would deposit a dollar or more into our account, have the savings book updated, and anticipate what we could do with over $50 when the holiday season came around.

"How about them Packers?"

So that was Green Bay in the 1950s, a working-class community dominated by families, neighborhoods, churches, and paper mills. Our city was like many others, except for one important detail. We had the Green Bay Packers. It's amazing that a city the size of Green Bay could have a professional sports team known all around the world. The community revolved around the Packers, which defined the city and its residents. It even gave people at a loss for words a fallback line, "How about them Packers?"

For many years, the Packers played their games in City Stadium with a seating capacity of around 25,000 fans. When the team moved to its current location at Lambeau Field, the number of seats increased considerably. The team needed to find a way to sell all those extra tickets. Our family was rather prominent in the community and stepped in to purchase several sets of season tickets.

In those days, the players lived in the same neighborhoods as the fans and promoted the team around the community. "Big John" Martinkovic was the closest any of us kids had ever been to a real Packer player. He lived over the garage of our backyard neighbor and came to our home to deliver tickets to a kickoff dinner, marking the opening of the new season. The event was heralded in the local paper, photo included, the proud fans with their adoring children in their matching shirts, sewn just for the occasion.

While the grownups used the season tickets, the kids attended games in a special children's section where a ticket cost one dollar. I still remember a fan who always sat right in front of the kids' section and who had the loudest voice I had ever heard. Other fans would often drink to excess, often starting at a tailgate party before the game. This led to many arguments and fights especially between Packer fans and those cheering for the archrival Chicago Bears.

Packer fans rarely gave up their season tickets and our family was no exception with the fourth generation attending games with those original Packer tickets. If a person wanted to apply for season tickets today, they would find themselves behind about 130,000 other eager fans with an approximate waiting time of thirty years.

Diversity

Green Bay in the 1960s was a White, working-class community where diversity and multiculturalism referred to someone who didn't cheer for the Packers. Predominantly Catholic and Lutheran, the residents were mostly from northern European backgrounds: Germans, Poles, Czechs, and Belgians with a large number of English and Irish descendants as well. In high school, I had a classmate whose family was from Mexico, the only person I knew who spoke any Spanish or any other language. Some Native American people lived within the city, chiefly on the near west side, but most lived on nearby reservations. About the only Black people in our community played for the Packers, though they had trouble finding people to rent to them in our homogeneous community. The nearest Blacks in my world lived in Milwaukee where I first saw billboards advertising hair care products to the Black population. The Great Migration of African Americans from the South to the cities of the North and West apparently stopped when it reached North Avenue in Milwaukee.

Dad used to take several of us down to Milwaukee to explore the museum or to visit one of his electronics friends. This was a time before the age of computers when electronics were first becoming popular. Dad embraced ham radio and let us listen to him talk to people all around the world with the home-built ham radio setup situated in our basement. "W9LON calling. I read you Brazil, Mexico or wherever." At his friend's electronics store, Dad inspected the inventory; we kids were admonished to keep out of trouble. The reward for not breaking anything would be a trip to Dad's favorite Chinese restaurant. He typically ordered his favorite pu pu platter and moo goo gai pan and then instructed us in the art of eating Chinese food with chopsticks. It wouldn't be long before these dinners with Dad would take on a new meaning.

My parents made it clear that our home wasn't just a place for our family alone. They set an example of hospitality for us by welcoming others into our home. They hosted church groups and Bible studies long before these were to become a common practice. One notable example of their attitude toward people different from us took place after Mom and Dad had gone out one evening. An African American musician had performed at a local supper club but was then refused dinner on account of his color. Dad invited him and his trio to have their dinner at our home.

Sometimes, I wonder how we all made it through childhood intact. Mary Barbara drove the car into the garage door. Lora put her arm through a glass door. Luke had a severe allergic reaction and required emergency treatment at home. I had an unfortunate run in with electricity. I was in kindergarten and, after lunch, had made a small car out of a blanket. Of course, a car needed a key to get started, so I found one for my vehicle. That got a little boring after a while until I got the idea that I could turn an electrical socket on with a key. I was almost electrocuted but only suffered burns on my hands, the first of many trips to St Vincent Hospital.

Looking back, I had a happy childhood in a loving home and a stable neighborhood in a safe community. I never knew anything but an environment where kids lived with their parents surrounded by family, church, neighbors, and friends. This was our world, and it didn't include people from other backgrounds, religions, or family settings. Single parents were likely to have lost their spouse and people felt sorry for children from "broken homes." My only contact with the word divorce would have come from some religion class or the rare mention of my mom's brother who actually married a divorced woman. Gasp! We never saw much of him. Who would have guessed we would soon have something in common with that long-lost uncle?

Chapter 3

Religion and Living by the Rules

When I was a child, I spoke as a child, I thought like a child, I'd reasoned like a child.

1 Corinthians 13:11a (ESV)

Spitballs from the choir loft

Growing up in a devout Catholic family meant religion was an ever-present reality of life. My parents were devoted to their Catholic faith and Dad had even attended a seminary for one year. He might even have gone on to become a priest but fortunately for me and my 13 siblings, the priesthood and celibacy weren't meant for him. Attending Catholic schools, we memorized the rules of the Church and learned to follow them, or else.

One Sunday morning, the four boys walked to St. Philip's to attend Sunday mass by ourselves. Our family usually sat in the front row in full view of the whole church. (I think this was one of Mom's strategies to keep us in line.) Without Mom's supervision, we were free to sneak up to the choir loft in the rear of the church, a forbidden activity. Undetected by the unsuspecting ushers and the people attending the Mass, we made little spitballs out of the Sunday bulletin and launched the paper projectiles toward various targets below, a man's hat, a lady's purse, the holy water font. We resisted the temptation to go for the man with the shiny bald head.

We joked about our little adventure on the way home from church until Joe announced, "You boys are in trouble for shooting spitballs in church." He confidently assured us that he had refrained from our spiritually deficient entertainment. The fear of consequences was great for Mark, John, and me, so we formulated a coverup plan. We had to keep this from our mother's attention. Our solution involved paying off Joe by taking him to DeLeers grocery store, conveniently located right on the way home from church. We all agreed this would be the perfect solution. We felt we were in the clear after buying Joe ice cream and candy, but our hopes were soon dashed.

Immediately upon our arrival at home, Joe proudly blurted out, "Mom, the boys were shooting spitballs from the choir loft at Mass today. And then, they went shopping on Sunday." We had engaged in two forbidden activities on a single Sunday morning! With this evidence of the waywardness of her sons, Mom compelled Mark, Johnny and me to march back to church to confess our transgression to the dreaded Monsignor who founded the parish, the one who actually interrupted the distribution of communion to call out people leaving early. I'm sure Mom wondered how this could have happened. Hadn't she trained us to join her nightly kneeling in the living room to pray the rosary? Where had she gone wrong? Years later, I would ask where I had gone wrong when my own children acted out in far worse ways at church.

It was one thing to confess our sins to the scowling Monsignor in the dark privacy of the confessional. That was uncomfortable, but at least he couldn't see us. To stand before him and confess in person was terrifying. We waited as he finished his lunch before we fearfully reported our behavior to him. I'm not sure what our punishment was but facing the Monsignor was more than enough punishment. For us, this was one step removed from appearing before the final judgment seat of God Himself.

The Four Boys continue to smile at the mention of our brush with eternal judgment. Mark, Johnny, and I still speak of Joe's restraint in the choir loft, but we credit Joe with telling Mom the truth. Telling the truth was a cardinal virtue in our home even if it takes a while. Almost 60 years after that day in the choir loft, Joe called me to confess that he too had joined in the spitball shooting. He wanted the truth to be known and felt he had to make restitution for his ill-gotten gains at the grocery store. We figured that with interest, penalties, and punitive damages, the amount would be substantial. But then, how does one report this on their taxes? And what about the potential trauma from our encounter with the monsignor?

Following the rules

Living by the Ten Commandments formed the basis for the development of my conscience and mine was very strong. Fear of eternal punishment can have that effect. My greatest sins included a brush with grand larceny (stealing 5 cents from a store), knocking the head off of a statue of Mary while playing ball in our classroom, and once writing a bad word on a chalkboard.

The Catholic Church had its own set of rules to be followed. One of the chief of these was the strict prohibition of eating meat on Fridays. One Friday, I was enjoying a Chicken-in-a-Biscuit cracker when a thought occurred to me. Did the name of the cracker suggest that it might contain some forbidden meat? I scrutinized the ingredient list and discovered to my horror that chicken was listed near the bottom. I should have suspected as much. Like Adam and Eve in the Garden, I had given into temptation and would be judged guilty. Another trip to the confessional for me.

This rule-based understanding of God strongly influenced my approach to other areas of life. I needed to have the good in my life outweigh the bad so I could get into heaven. Through attendance at Catholic grade school and high school, I developed the unshakable assurance that it was through the Catholic Church that I could find my way into heaven. God was someone to be respected and feared, and religion was about doing the right things for others to see. Missing from this was any personal conviction that faith itself is a gift from God.

With my emphasis on doing the right things, I served as an altar boy to assist at Mass and later was appointed youth representative to the parish council. Recognizing my interest in church related matters, my mother even entertained the idea that I might become a priest, though I wasn't too excited, even though I had been born on a feast day celebrating Mary.

My Catholic upbringing equipped me with a strong moral foundation and sense of conscience. The Church provided a tremendous sense of security and bound together the other parts of my life. There could be little question about the difference between right and wrong and how people were supposed to act. I was certain that the people around me would live by these rules too. How wrong I was. The grownups in my life were secretly taking a different path from the one they talked about on Sunday. My confidence in the power of religion to protect me was about to be broken.

Chapter 4

The Family Unravels; the Search for Answers Begins

God sets the lonely in families.

Psalm 68:6 (NIV)

Where's Dad?

Sometime after my tenth birthday, I began to realize that our family life was changing. Up to that point, my biggest concern was the 1960 presidential election. Young, handsome war hero John F Kennedy was running to become the first Catholic president ever! With his beautiful wife and young children, his family was a model of the American dream. I stayed up watching TV late into the night to watch the election returns. It all came down to Illinois, the last state to be decided, and there was no way I could go to sleep until the winner was declared. We celebrated the next day at school. Years later came my rude awakening to the realities of national politics. People joked that the election took so long to be decided because they had trouble counting the votes cast in Chicago's cemetery precincts.

We were elated and celebrated his victory at home and at school. When the new president challenged citizens to look for the greater good of the country at his inauguration, "Ask not what your country can do for you. Ask what you can do for your country," I imagined myself entering the dream world of Camelot. All was well in my world.

The real world at home was a different matter, a different kind of dream, one where we began to ask different questions. "Where's Dad this morning? Did he make it home last night? Where did that bottle of Southern Comfort come from? What was all that yelling about last night?" Sequestered in our basement bedrooms, we knew something bad was going on upstairs but had no idea of its significance.

I knew Dad worked long hours and often had emergencies to take care of through the night. A busy doctor could always find good reasons to be somewhere they would rather be than at home. I didn't realize Dad was starting to sleep on a new bed, a bench in the doctors' lounge at the hospital, and not just so he could take care of his patients. At first, we thought he needed to be there to take care of sick patients, but now, he seemed to be gone more.

Then life changed in a way I could never have imagined. It was Good Friday, and we spent the afternoon in the long, solemn service with the church statues draped in black to remind us of the sadness of that day. I didn't need any reminders when I returned home to a scene even more somber; Dad had moved out. He wouldn't be sleeping at home anymore and life would never be the same. No more reading in bed. No more riding with him on house calls or to Milwaukee or to visit Grandma's house. No more Camelot on Louise Street.

To people outside our family, our family life probably appeared to be going well, but we knew there were problems. My parents had begun arguing with greater frequency and verbal intensity, with an occasional slammed door provided for emphasis. We kids huddled in the basement as our parents verbally assaulted each other. (Decades later, one of my siblings shared the haunting thought that maybe things might have turned out differently if we children had confronted our parents about their fighting. But of course, we never did, in an era when children were seen, not heard.)

Decades later, Mom shared that troubles had started in the years after Susie's death. Mom dealt with her grief by turning to Southern Comfort. The problems with drinking eventually worsened to the point that Dad had her admitted to the Brown County Mental Health Center for treatment.

While Mom was hospitalized, Mary Barbara decided to have a few friends over to our house. I doubt she realized that her little get together would take place on the very night Mom was to be released from the hospital. Word got out about the cozy gathering and soon our house was filled with partying teenagers. An upset neighbor called the police. Imagine my mother's shock when my parents pulled into the driveway after her discharge from the hospital.

Police cars surrounded our house, and officers were rounding up the partying teens. We younger kids had been sent downstairs before the party but were now called on to shelter some of the fleeing couples in our bedrooms. I was twelve or thirteen and couldn't imagine that these teen couples weren't uncomfortable in a crib or under a bed or in a closet together. How could they breathe under all those blankets? It didn't occur to me that they had other things on their minds.

Dad was able to smooth things over with the police but the hospitalization and party changed the atmosphere around the house. I doubt if any of us realized at the time what an involuntary commitment meant to the person being hospitalized against their will. The loss of autonomy and freedom would be painful for anyone in this situation. How much more so when the commitment was sought by the patient's spouse? The hospitalization brought Mom's alcoholism out into the open, no longer able to be denied or ignored, least of all in a family with thirteen children. As far as I understood it, Mom never drank again after that stay in the hospital.

Within the next year or so, Lucy, my youngest sister, was born. Problems at home worsened to the point that Nancy was sent to live with Grandma and Grandpa Warpinski for a school year. Nobody ever talked about why she was sent away. A few years later, when Nancy and Margaret tried to run away to Grandma's house, Mom tracked them down and sent Dad to retrieve them. Dad found them on their way and brought them home (after taking them out to lunch at their favorite restaurant.) My parents had different views on discipline and childrearing.

After his Good Friday departure, Dad eventually rented a house close to my paper route. I started sneaking down to his place after delivering my papers. The house was empty and quiet; I can't recall Dad ever being there during one of my clandestine visits. I could read or listen to music like *Take 5* by the Dave Brubeck quartet or something by the Beatles who were fast becoming the musical rage. On the couch in Dad's living room, eyes closed, listening to the Beatles or the Dave Brubeck quartet, I was free from commotion and fighting. Who could ask for more?

In one sense, my parents' separation had some positive impact on my life, but it never meant getting twice as many Christmas presents.

The solitude at Dad's was scant consolation. He was never around to enjoy it with. From this time on, we only saw Dad in accordance with the court-ordered visitation schedule which meant at his discretion and with a twenty-four hour notification. He rarely made the call.

Dad's new arrangement worked for a while, but social conventions in the 1960s were strict and unbending. This was years before no-fault divorce laws made getting a divorce easier to obtain and, in some cases, even without the consent of both spouses. Obtaining a divorce in Wisconsin without evidence of domestic violence or infidelity was out of the question and the Catholic Church was clear in its prohibition of divorce as well. The social pressure made medical practice and life in general increasingly uncomfortable for him. He left his clinic and opened a new office next door to an orthodontist. I had my braces started there but only the upper teeth straightened by the time Dad left town altogether and my remaining appointments were canceled. My bottom teeth are still crooked, a daily reminder of how Dad's departure affected my teenage years.

In those days, social norms were clear. A man with a wife and thirteen children just didn't leave them behind and move on to a new life. As a final desperate move to save our family, Mom challenged Dad about his plans. That's when she loaded us up for that fateful day at Dad's office. Some time passed after the lineup before Dad moved to Las Vegas to complete the divorce proceedings. The next day he married MaryAnn, a nurse he had worked with in Green Bay. They would go on to have Cecelia and Anastasia, two more sisters, strangers to me for most of my life, another unmentionable topic around our house. Decades later, we have finally gotten to know and appreciate each other as adults.

The family I grew up in would never be united again. Joe moved out to Las Vegas with Dad, and I had only occasional contact with him for years. My siblings and I still talk about the reasons for Joe's departure and whether Dad tried to gain custody of the rest of us. Around the time Dad left, Mary Barbara and Kathy moved out of the house to pursue school, travel, and work. This left Mark, the oldest of the remaining children at home, to be Mom's right-hand man and me as his lieutenant until he left for college a few years later.

I see Grandma's house

We gradually lost touch with Dad's side of the family, the grandparents, aunts, uncles, and cousins. But for us kids, the most tangible loss was the food we looked forward to sharing on our visits to Grandma and Grandpa's house in the country. As we neared their home, each of the kids would anxiously strain to be the first to spy their house off in the distance and call out, "I see Grandma's house!"

Grandma specialized in frying fresh donuts and tossing them with sugar in a brown paper grocery bag. As we rushed into the house, the irresistible aroma of the donuts drew us into Grandma's inviting kitchen. Warm and filled with raisins and covered with sugar, the donuts disappeared as quickly as Grandma could produce them for the hungry children clamoring for yet another donut from her fryer.

We didn't have quite the same enthusiasm for her other signature dish, Czarnina (pronounced ched-knee-na), also known as Polish duck blood soup. In case the reader might have trouble finding the recipe, the procedure went something like this. Grandpa would slaughter a duck and collect the blood. Grandma would roast the duck and cook it up into a soup with its blood, raisins, vinegar, sugar, and dumplings. We would all have to try a little of this delicacy, and I still get shivers when I think of that sweet, vinegary blood soup. (I learned recently that this popular Eastern European food has a special meaning. According to one account, unsuccessful Polish suitors might receive some *Czarnina* from the maiden's parents. This let him know that he had been unsuccessful in his pursuit of their daughter.) It's interesting that at our family reunions, several of my cousins still try to replicate Grandma's donut recipe, but I can't recall anyone ever making the effort to produce more *Czarnina*. For some foods, it's probably best to be content with the memory. And let sleeping ducks lie.

Off limits

With Dad's leaving, major changes took place at home. My parents' bedroom had always been their private sanctuary. We kids were virtually never allowed in there. On rare occasions, Mom would give us specific instructions to retrieve some item from the bedroom. We were to leave the room immediately and not look around, like Lot's wife before she was turned into a pillar of salt. Was there some potential hazard awaiting us should we spend too much time there? But how could I resist taking a moment to look at Dad's bed and recall that wonderful time when I read to him many years earlier. Probably best not to think about it too much. Eventually, to keep us from sneaking into the room, Mom began locking the door, freezing it in place, our family's own time capsule.

Mom abandoned the master bedroom and moved across the hall. Were the memories from her own bedroom just too painful for her to bear? Gradually, the bedroom filled with clothing, household goods and grocery bags full of boxes of Chex cereal and cans of peanuts. Harkening back to her Bohemian heritage, Mom developed a reputation for making "Czech" party mix. This soon became one of our family traditions, the iconic food we all share at family gatherings.

Later, Mom appropriated the third upstairs bedroom, replacing the crib with a hospital bed which she felt gave her better sleep. I don't recall her ever being seriously ill, though she would commonly retreat to the hospital bed with some comment like "I think it's my ticker. I don't think I'm perking like I used to." We would simply let her be until she was revived and ready for more of our family life.

Life with a single parent

Mom was under constant pressure to run the entire household with kids ranging from infancy to high school. Not only did she need to keep us all cooperating with each other (as in the morning rush for a shower), she had to make sure we all got out the door on time. She developed some novel strategies to accomplish this. "Milk is on the cereal!" Mom would call down to our basement barracks each school morning. We scrambled up the stairs to grab our cornflakes and hunt for a place to sit. A moment's delay meant hopelessly soggy corn flakes awaited us.

When the divorce was finalized, our family lived in a state of continual financial stress, always hoping the child support money would arrive on time as ordered by the courts. I couldn't begin to count how many times Mom called the Clerk of Courts office to see if the support check arrived as scheduled only to be disappointed once again. She would have to make do for another week. And so would the rest of us. That's when Mom relied on our babysitting money to make ends meet; my younger siblings tell me they babysat for over thirty families and cleaned rooms at school to pay for their high school tuition. When they were old enough to get jobs, that money also went to support the family. Only when they turned eighteen could they keep their earnings for themselves.

I resented the inconsistent flow of child support because of the strain it put on Mom. I eventually had it out with MaryAnn years later. I had always believed she was behind the delayed payments, and I pressed her to explain why the checks were late, time after time. Was the money just not available or was this just another way of pressuring Mom over some adult issue? I still don't know. I only knew we were always in suspense over when the check would arrive.

I wonder why I never asked my dad this question or any of the other countless questions I had about growing up under these circumstances. Was I afraid to call him out on this or more likely, was I afraid of the answer I might get? Safer to attribute this to my middle child status than as one who avoids confrontation.

Fortunately, Mom and the rest of us at home were supported by extended family, our parish, and the community, with food baskets and holiday meals dropped off at our home during times of particular need. Aunts and uncles on Mom's side practically adopted us at times for extended sleepovers, and countless meals. We rarely saw anyone on Dad's side of the family unless he was in town. No one ever told us why. During the vegetable harvest season, we followed the trucks to the canning plant hoping to collect peas jarred off the truck by the bumpy road. I understood that financial security could only come through my own efforts.

The effects of Dad's departure extended far beyond the financial. Gone were all the radio and electronics gear. There were no more army surplus treasures, no more trips to Milwaukee, and no more exposure to the local medical community or to classical music like Dad's favorite opera *la Traviata*. Gone was someone who knew me well enough to guide me through the teenage years.

These are all things someone on the outside could observe. It's harder to describe what it's like to descend from our lofty status in the community to become the subject of gossip and recipients of handouts. This reversal of fortune could easily have broken many people but not my mother. She related a story of once being at church where two women were gossiping about her and our family. They were speaking in Bohemian not realizing that that was her native language growing up. Imagine their shock when she greeted them with perfect inflection.

By the time I was a sophomore in high school, all my older siblings had moved out of the house to pursue school or work. I became the de facto "Man of the House" and for the next several years, felt it my responsibility to look out for Mom and my younger siblings. It seemed like my mother and my sisters were frequently at odds with each other while we boys got along pretty well with her. I found myself in the position of family mediator. Someone had to represent them when they had a hard time getting Mom to understand their troubles and concerns.

With so many children and only one car, Mom had to seriously curtail our outside activities at school and in the community. There was no way she could have driven us around to lessons or other activities apart from school and church. She did drive me to grade school basketball tournaments with my teammates, conscripting us to pray the rosary with her on the way to the game. Just what every thirteen-year-old boy wanted to do.

I still wish I could have gotten involved in scouting but was prevented by the lack of transportation and funds. Our family had once been well-respected in the community and even rather prosperous. My parents had once traveled to Cuba for a vacation and took the four boys to Chicago and Washington DC. Now we had no disposable income and no longer took any more family trips. Each of the kids had to work if they wanted to have any spending money for clothing or the other necessities of teenage life.

Uncomfortable topic

As a child, it never dawned on me that my parents' bedroom would be for anything other than sleeping or reading. Given the fact that Dad fathered fourteen children, they must have used the bed for something more than that. My sister, Nancy, once told me a story when she was learning about the birds and the bees and came to realize that. She was shocked when a cousin said that with fourteen children in our family, our parents had "done it" that many times. Nancy's angry response was to punch the cousin in the stomach. End of discussion. We never talked about sex in our household. Like politics or just about anything related to Dad, it was a forbidden subject. I would have to learn about sex on my own.

Unfortunately, with no older siblings around, I was left to fend for myself when it came to answering questions important to a teenage boy. I was probably a little slow in coming to understand things related to the opposite sex. I recall my mother once assuring me that if I ever had any questions about "certain things," I could always talk to Uncle Paul. I thanked her for that offer but was puzzled about what kind of things she was actually referring to. It was quite a while later that I came to realize she was talking about *those* kinds of things. Knowing that wouldn't have mattered; I was too embarrassed to talk to Uncle Paul in any case.

Entering seventh or eighth grade, I still didn't have much of an understanding of why boys would show an interest in girls. I was uncomfortable around girls and at times unkind to some of my female classmates mostly with hurtful words. This kind of bullying is something I still regret, even decades later. On the other hand, some of the boys in my class were definitely more advanced in their amorous pursuits. We had all been thoroughly warned by our teacher, a Catholic nun, that close contact with the opposite sex was certain to be a serious sin. She admonished us that if you couldn't slip a thin butter knife between a boy and girl who were dancing, they were almost certainly in the act of committing a grave sin. It never occurred to me to ask what the dance partners would be doing with a butter knife on the dance floor. Probably a good thing, as asking such an impertinent question would likely have led to getting kicked out of school a third time.

Catholic grade schools at the time were notoriously strict; getting rapped on the knuckles with a ruler or pinched on the ear wasn't at all uncommon. Discipline reigned. In fourth grade, I was in a third/fourth grade split. The teacher was talking to the third graders about fractions and dividing objects like apples or oranges. A student asked her how one could divide things like pencils. The frustrated teacher explained that some things couldn't be divided. With my advanced understanding of mathematics, I took a pencil from my desk, held it over my head and snapped it in two, gaining the attention of my classmates. The teacher, however, was not amused by this helpful demonstration and sent me to the office, my first suspension from school. With a family our size, having one of us in the office wasn't unusual. They could have used a speed dial had it been available. My mother had to come get me reinstated.

Several years later, suspension resulted when I whispered to a friend during music class. I was afraid to go home that day and instead, hid among the altar boy vestments in church until I finally summoned enough courage to make my dreaded report to Mom. Times have certainly changed as I now think about what it would take to get suspended from school today. I'm confident it would be a lot more than breaking a pencil or whispering in class.

Fortunately, I didn't always get caught while causing trouble, like the time we had an indoor lunch recess and were bowling in our classroom. A little too much spin caused the ball to bounce off of a desk and into a statue in the devotional area of the classroom. Another trip to confession for me, this time for decapitating the blessed Virgin.

My interest in coin collecting was also at the root of the first crime I committed. The love of money truly is the root of all evil. In those days, a person could find valuable coins by searching through rolls of coins for rare specimens. One time, I obtained a roll of forty nickels for $2.00. After removing the Indian Head nickels, steel nickels and rare dates, I put only thirty-nine nickels back in the roll and kept one for myself. Almost immediately after exchanging the roll at a store, I was conscience-stricken. How could I bear to keep that nickel in my possession? I was too embarrassed to go back to the store and admit that I had stolen five cents. What could I do? I solved my dilemma by sneaking over to the nearby pizza parlor. With nobody looking, I buried the nickel in the planter by the entrance. From that point on, I resolved to never take something that didn't belong to me even if I could get away with it. When I found a dime in church one day, my conscience wouldn't let me keep it, so I used the coin to light a votive candle.

One evening in eighth grade, my friend and I were over at a girl's house when her mother was away. My friend and one of the girls somehow found themselves locked into a bedroom closet. I sat on the bed trying to figure out a way to rescue them from their imprisonment. They assured me that they were going to be okay in the closet and that I shouldn't worry. They would be safe until they found a way out. Meanwhile, the other girl started getting a little too close for my comfort. I managed to put her dog between us to maintain a safe distance between us (more than enough for our teacher's "butter knife" rule.) Thankfully, my friend and the other girl survived their ordeal in the closet without any noticeable adverse effect. I never actually kissed a girl until well into my high school years, and, even then, it was not a comfortable experience for me.

Seeking approval

After Dad moved to Las Vegas, he would return to Green Bay about once a year until his mother passed away. While he was home, we would all get to see him over dinner at a restaurant. It's hard to imagine what it's like when up to ten kids are having their annual audience with their dad, seated around a long dining table, each one vying for his attention. Dad would try to ask each of us how we were doing, but the conversation really turned into a matter of us answering in ways that might make us stand out in the crowd.

The competition for Dad's approval was intense as each of us reported on our grades or anything that we thought might make him proud. To us, it was all about having something of value to report, some new accomplishment, something that would make us stand out. I'm sure these attempts to impress Dad became part of my way of relating to other people. (It's interesting to note that fifty years later, my siblings and I now meet for weekly Zoom calls. One might think that this type of sibling rivalry and vying for attention would have ended by now for each of us has achieved success in life. Not the case. The oldest ones in each cohort still take centerstage, the middle ones are still in the audience. All seated around a virtual dinner table with Dad, present in spirit thirty years after his passing, at the head patiently receiving the next round of progress reports.)

The competition between my siblings and I wasn't only about getting Dad's attention. We also wanted to look best in Mom's eyes as well. There was an ongoing debate about which one of the kids was Mom's favorite. We frequently argued at home about which one of the kids she loved most. This took an amusing turn on one occasion when some writing was discovered on the inside of a basement cabinet stating, "John hates Mom. Signed John." No one would admit who tried to set Johnny up.

The positives start to appear

From my teenage years and well into my adult life, I could only see the negative aspects of my parents' divorce and the challenges and disappointments of life. I grieved over my own painful loss of connection with my dad's side of the family. I resented the shortage of resources in our household and the fact that I had to work to put myself through school. My friends had a dad around the house, and I didn't.

I didn't realize it at the time, but something good was going to come from the contrasting choices my parents made. While Dad drove several days across the country to start his new life, Mom drove across town to join her brother Paul for weekly Alcoholics Anonymous meetings. Mom spent the next 50 years as an active member of AA, sponsoring many others in their attempts to overcome alcoholism. She also took my younger siblings to Alateen meetings for children of alcoholics. Overcoming alcoholism, rejection and abandonment, Mom built a new life as a single parent.

In the Book of Proverbs, there is a passage about the model woman who demonstrates faithfulness, hard work, and devotion to her family, the very attributes I saw in my mother. Of course, she wasn't perfect. We all have our shortcomings, but I'm sure I would have many more if it hadn't been for her example.

It would be years before I could acknowledge that my early life experiences shaped me for a successful life journey. I had learned firsthand the cost of being a faithful parent who puts their children before their personal desires. There is no question that my mother was responsible for raising our family and she is the one to whom we owe the greatest debt. Our family was also supported by countless others, often without my knowledge, unsung heroes who made my personal success more attainable.

But the negative consequences of alcoholism and parental divorce would dominate my thinking well into my adult life. My faulty thinking would lead me to make many poor choices and mistakes of my own. The three interlocking dimensions of my early life: middle child, alcoholism, and divorce became the basis for how I would approach life. They would influence patterns of communication that would lead to future problems, but I didn't know that at the time. My attention was directed toward being a loyal son and successful student preparing to embark on a life journey of his own outfitted with the right knowledge, skills, and abilities. These would require years of education and training. I would be on my own, free to risk loving and trusting another without fear of being abandoned but without Dad's guidance.

Divorce affects all areas of a child's life regardless of how hard the parents try to have that not be the case. Some people even say the children of divorce can be better off. After all, they say, happy parents lead to happy children. I would disagree, except in cases of physical or emotional abuse. The real message of divorce is that all of life's commitments are conditional, honored only as long as both partners see the marriage being to their advantage. No one ever asks the children about their wishes, as if they could possibly know what was in store for them. All I know is that for me, my family dissolved as I entered my teen years, a time when patterns of thinking and behavior are becoming established. I was developing some unhealthy patterns and lived much of my life in the fallout of the choices my parents had made.

Chapter 5

Equipped for Life's Journey

Trust in the Lord with all your heart and lean not on your own understanding; in all your ways submit to him and he will make your paths straight.

Proverbs 3: 5- 6 (NIV)

My son, obey your father's commands, and don't neglect your mother's instruction.

Proverbs 6:20 (NLT)

Student for life

"What do you want to be when you grow up?" I asked my young patient just like I had been asked many times growing up.

"I want to be a doctor," he confidently replied.

"Do you like school?"

"Not really. I can't wait until I'm done."

"How long do you think it takes to become a doctor?"

"I don't know, ten or twelve years?"

"Actually, that will get you about halfway there. It usually takes at least 11 years after high school, although for some, like me, it takes longer. I hope you start liking school soon."

School can be a great place for someone who craves attention and recognition. While no one told me it would take almost twenty-five years of education to become a doctor, I'm not sure that would have discouraged me. I simply loved being in school and learning. Given my family background, this probably wouldn't be much of a surprise. Both of my parents placed a high value on education. Along with my older siblings, they set a high bar for grades and other achievements. Getting a good report card became one of my main goals in life. Each A was worth one dollar, a generous amount at a time when a bottle of soda cost ten cents. Few things could top straight A's.

School came easily and provided opportunities to compete for recognition through extra credit work, projects, and answering questions in class. I must have taken this to an extreme like the day I raised my hand so often that I risked a rotator cuff injury. The teacher forbade me from answering any more questions for an entire day. My classmates also needed a chance to speak.

Each of the kids in our family sought to distinguish themselves in some way. For one, it might be in music or the arts; for another, it was sports, but for me, it was always going to be academics. We each had the opportunity to attend Catholic high school. Even if our family was poor in financial terms, there was never any doubt about Dad supporting my private education through high school. (Years later, I learned that my younger siblings weren't so fortunate and had to work to help pay for their high school education.) Nor was there any question about what kinds of students we would associate with. Beginning in grade school, I surrounded myself with high achievers. For fun, we would get together on the weekends to make homemade pizzas and talk about homework and sports. Girls never entered the discussion.

The college-prep orientation of our school outlined a course of study based on the results of the student's entrance test. For those in the top cohort, that meant four years of foreign languages, starting with two years of Latin. As an aspiring doctor, that was fine with me, even though one of my Latin teachers was the strictest teacher I had ever experienced. On the first day of class, he laid out the rules of engagement for the class. Students had twenty-three other hours of the day to cough, sneeze, or go to the bathroom. After completing two years of Latin, my friends and I decided to take Russian, considered to be the most difficult language offered at the school. I loved learning about Russian history, culture, and literature and still enjoy listening to the lyrical Russian language. On the other hand, certain classes such as art, woodworking, and shop were off limits for students in my group. Some of my friends learned this at home, but not me.

In addition to the academics, our school offered ROTC (Reserve Officers Training Corps) which taught me discipline and responsibility and gave me a favorable impression of the military. The training included target practice for which I was to be awarded a ribbon for my marksmanship abilities. My fame was short-lived, however, when the cadet next to me was mistakenly aiming at my target; between us we had scored enough points on my target to merit an award. So much for my marksmanship recognition. Over 50 years after my graduation, I was speaking with a group of students at my alma mater about my high school experiences. They were shocked and frightened to think that there could be a firing range in a school. Another indication of the sheltered life I was blessed with.

I aspired to become a "Renaissance Man" accomplished in many different areas even if not the best at any of them. Several of my classmates and I competed with some success against other high school students on Five High, a local television program. The show was modeled after The College Bowl which was popular on TV at the time. Students competed by answering questions about obscure facts and relatively unknown bits of information. Just right for someone like me, who passed his free time reading encyclopedias and looking up words in dictionaries. No activity was beyond my interest including sports such as track and intramural basketball, different school clubs, and volunteer activities in the community. Service at church involved being the student representative on the parish council.

Our family often sang in city talent shows, as though we had come right out of the *Sound of Music*. I loved music and even sang and danced in the school musical, but I never pursued music studies. Life was busy, and we couldn't afford piano lessons, so I followed my brother Mark's lead and bought my first guitar. It didn't take long for my younger brother, Johnny, to pick it up and play with a skill that I was never able to attain. I ceded control of my guitar to him and only learned the basics after that, never really pursuing the instrument. What seemed like a small decision at the time turned out to set up a pattern for the future. Determined to be seen as a success, I often dropped out of activities I had enjoyed to avoid failure. It wasn't good enough to simply enjoy an activity. I had to be the best or else find something else to do.

With such a large family crowded into our house, I would often look for somewhere to go to get away from all the commotion.

Sometimes, this meant spending school nights at my cousin Katie's house, which was closer to my school and definitely quieter than our noisy home environment. Staying there, I was also able to get up early before school to watch University of the Air programs. This became one of my favorite activities, an opportunity to learn about many new topics and learn more random information for my game show career. Staying with relatives was also another way in which my siblings and I were supported by the larger family of relatives looking out for us.

My learning wasn't limited to the classroom. When the park shelter closed at the end of summer, Mom had to find other ways to keep us occupied. My motivation to get out of the house was somewhat different. Complaining about boredom would likely earn the opportunity to do more chores. Mom's cure for our ennui was to drive several of us kids downtown on Saturday mornings and drop us off for several hours at the library and the museum which were both located in the same building. As a confirmed bookworm and museum lover, I couldn't have asked for a better arrangement. Out of the house and with no chores to do, I could explore the basement museum with its collection of countless objects of interest. When I'd had enough of the Egyptian mummy, Indian artifacts and the stuffed animals on display, I would proceed upstairs to the library. It was just like being in our living room, only bigger. In the solitude of the library, I could read to my heart's content. When we all had enough of the museum and library, we headed next door to a bowling alley for a few games. What present-day parent could drop off school-age kids downtown without incurring some sort of citation for negligence? Life in the 60's was more secure and less complicated.

Being pretty shy and uncomfortable around girls, I don't have many fond memories of dating in high school. My all-boys high school was affiliated with the all-girls Catholic school across town where my sisters attended. Our primary contact with the girls' school took place watching sporting events together, attending school dances, and participating in the school play. It's hard to imagine now what it might have been like to have girls in my classes, but at least I didn't have to worry about trying to impress them with my appearance or performance. On the other hand, having girls my age around in school would very likely have helped me develop more confidence in their presence. For me, contact with girls would largely be restricted to family life with my six younger sisters.

Starting around fourth grade, I began to get the sense that I was going to be a doctor or maybe a teacher though nobody in our house gave me much guidance either way. During high school, my thinking went back and forth until I discussed careers with a trusted teacher. "Choose medicine," he said without hesitation, "it's a much better career." That ended the questioning and I never looked at anything but medicine from then on. Nevertheless, I still loved the idea of being a teacher and looked for ways to teach in many different settings.

Nearing the end of high school, the question of where to attend college had to be addressed. I wanted to go to college close to home partly out of a sense of responsibility for my family but probably also out of anxiety about being completely out on my own. I didn't relish the thought of competing with large numbers of other students and decided I would rather try to distinguish myself in a smaller setting where I would have a greater chance of having something to share at the annual dinner with Dad.

The day after high school graduation, Dad drove Mark, Joe, Kathy, and me out to spend the summer with him and his new family in Las Vegas. To keep us all hydrated on the way, he filled an oversized thermos with some type of fruit punch. Each time we stopped for gas, he would fill up the thermos with water and ice, but he never added any more fruit punch. The tasty drink was deep red in Wisconsin, light pink in Nebraska and homeopathic-strength by the time we reached our final destination. I had never driven on an interstate before this time, but Dad gave me the duty of driving a night shift across Iowa. Since there weren't many cars on the road, I thought it was best to center my car on the dashed white line dividing the two lanes of westbound traffic. Why were all these cars honking their horns at me? Dad had been sleeping in the front seat and woke up startled. He took one look at my driving and made a comment that is probably best left out of print.

College: Looking for affirmation–from lab to rooftop to soccer field

Paying for college was going to pose new challenges to my financial security. My family only paid for one course of my entire college career. (Mark, Joe, and I took a class together at UNLV studying contemporary English drama. I had absolutely no background in the subject and won't say who got the highest grade. Suffice it to say, our intrinsic competitiveness spurred us all on in this class.) The rest of my college education was funded through scholarships and various jobs, something that's practically impossible these days.

Fortunately, I was awarded a scholarship to attend UW Green Bay which covered many of my basic needs. A work study job in the chemistry/physics department completed my financial aid package and changed the course of my college career.

The University of Wisconsin had just built a new campus in Green Bay, and mine would be the first class to attend in the newly constructed buildings. My job was to set up the labs and then do the experiments during the summer that other chemistry students would be doing in the fall. I was always one or two weeks ahead of the classes, but, as it turned out, I actually had to take these same classes for credit. My job provided a great way to get better at lab work, and it certainly helped my grades as well.

As a pre-med student, I felt a definite pressure to succeed in every college course I took. Early on, I was shocked to find that I was failing a required course in calculus. "Drop the class and take it again next year," advised the professor.

"I can't drop this class! it will throw off my entire pre-med course of study." I had never failed anything in school and couldn't imagine starting now. Though I received the lowest grade of my educational career, I passed the course and was able to stay on track with my plan to become a doctor.

Having such a definite long-range plan helped me maintain focus while developing the ability to put off enjoyable things in the present time for a long-term benefit. At the same time, I didn't realize at the time how much this attitude actually cost me. Although I was interested in history, art, and music, I took little more than the required courses in these subjects. On one occasion, I was taking an art class, and it appeared that I might not even be able to receive a B. Fearing the impact of a C on my GPA, I dropped the class, even though I enjoyed learning the material.

Since I worked for the school, I was also able to meet many of my future teachers and work for them in the lab. This opened up the opportunity to be student director of a National Science Foundation research project looking at the health effects of air pollution in our community. A second project looked for cancer-causing pollutants in the local air. Not everyone gets to admire the sunrise from the top of City Hall. Years later, I found myself back on the rooftop of the Madison Veterans Hospital to collect pollen samples as part of my allergy fellowship training. None of these lab and research experiences would have been possible had I not been forced to work my way through school.

Things didn't always work out quite so well with my job in the lab. Before school started the first semester, I was assigned the task of checking the emergency showers in each of the labs. I'd never seen a shower without a floor drain before and assumed I could simply hold a wastebasket over my head to collect the water when the shower was activated. How was I to know that an emergency shower in a lab dispenses a torrent of twenty-five gallons of water in a matter of seconds? I could have asked, but that would have suggested I didn't know. In trying to save face, I embarrassed myself in the process, leaving myself soaking wet. In any case, some would call this getting immersed in one's work.

My work in the labs also got me in closer contact with other teachers in the sciences, which led to new social opportunities. The chairperson of the biology department was having an evening get together at her waterfront home. I had never been to a professor's house before and was nervously eating potato chips and dip when she approached me. "How do you like that dip?" she inquired. "Okay, I guess," (which really meant it was the blandest, least flavorful chip dip I had ever eaten.) "Interesting," she remarked, "That's the whipped butter you're eating. The chip dip is over there."

Some of us are a little slower at learning social conventions than others. One evening, some friends and I went fishing for smelt during the spring spawning season. Smelt fishing involved catching large numbers of the small fish in the creeks off of Green Bay or Lake Michigan. Catching a couple of thousand smelt was the easy part. Next, they had to be cleaned. After staying up all night and cleaning and freezing the fish, we went right to class not anticipating the classroom response to our fishy smell.

There were no sports teams on campus when I started at UWGB. With football out of the question (the new school hardly had enough students to make up a team), soccer was the next best choice. The first order of business was to recruit some accomplished soccer players to form the nucleus of the team. Where would the school find the rest of the players to surround them? The most practical solution was to find interested local students and teach them how to play soccer, providing the star players a chance to succeed for the team to be respectable. I had never played soccer in my life but somehow found myself on the college soccer team. I had a lot of experience with distance running in high school, so I could at least keep up during all the practices. I was stationed as a defender where there would be other layers of defense to protect our goal, amazed that even a player with minimal talent and no experience could still get on the field. Playing college sports was another advantage of going to a small school. This experience came in handy later as I was able to coach my own children's soccer teams with some level of success, at least enough to allow them to play.

The combination of good grades, extracurricular activities and research projects made for a strong scholarship application for medical school. In the end, I was selected for a Health Professions Scholarship: Four years of medical school tuition and money for living expenses in return for four years of service in the US Air Force. I had enjoyed ROTC and looked forward to even more of the camaraderie and structure that would come with full time service. And I could avoid going deeply into debt to pay for medical school

Being mostly on my own at this point in life did have some challenging aspects as well. Before I realized and accepted how harmful drinking had been in my family's life, I followed the path of many of my classmates with underage drinking. I still remember the time we managed to get a fifth of Southern Comfort and hide it at my grandmother's house until we could have a little party. When the time for our party came, my friends and I went back to retrieve our treasure only to be greatly disappointed. The Southern Comfort was nowhere to be found. Two of my uncles had discovered it. While I didn't recognize it at the time, I was at risk of following in my mother's footsteps into alcohol abuse. My uncles had spared me of at least one drinking episode. But that wasn't enough to get me to stop drinking altogether. That came in stages, starting with the high school graduation party when I was too drunk to come to the door to see my mother who had come to wish me well before I left with my dad for the summer. (Another drinking episode settled the matter of drinking several years later when I had too much to drink while out with one of my medical school preceptors. I ended up sleeping through dinner.)

To support myself in high school and college, I worked a variety of jobs besides the lab as illustrated in these vignettes:

Managing a drive-in restaurant

Summer employment during high school involved working about sixty miles from home at a drive-in restaurant in Door County. Without a car, I often hitchhiked when I couldn't find a more predictable ride. Owned and operated by my high school English teacher and his wife, the drive-in catered to the local clientele and tourists during the afternoon and evening hours. At night, we served seasonal workers on the upper Midwest fruit and vegetable-picking circuit–peaches and blueberries in Michigan, cherries in Door County, vegetables in southern Wisconsin, then back to the south for winter work.

This was my first exposure to people who spoke Spanish. I wondered about these men. Who were they? Where did they and their families live? About the only thing I learned about them was that they liked deep-fried shrimp.

My coworker was a high school classmate, and together we did much of the cooking and ran the restaurant for the evening shift. One of us was designated Assistant Drive-in Manager while the other had the title Associate Drive-in Manager. We never could decide which of us had a higher ranking. It didn't matter. The job was a great opportunity to learn about business and take responsibility. And I now had my first professional title. As a bonus, the owner even gave us English lessons and assignments for no extra charge.

When I wasn't managing the drive-in, I picked up extra work in a nearby cherry orchard where I learned enough to consider myself an expert on horticulture. And did I mention I was required to take turns babysitting the owner's four kids?

Summer in Door County wasn't only about the job. On one occasion, I was attempting to talk to the girl living next door to the drive-in. It was late and I couldn't just go to the door, so I climbed the tree outside her window. *Pretty daring,* I thought, *just like in some story of romance.* Just as I reached my destination, the romance switched to reality by the girl's shotgun-waving father. Back to the deep fryer for me.

Life in the real world

After high school, I worked in Las Vegas for two summers, a naive, trusting Midwestern boy in a world of fast living and quick riches, where the highways had no speed limits and neither did life. Dad's neighbor pulled some strings to land me a job as a busboy at the

Riviera, then a prestigious hotel on the Strip. That was it. My main qualification for the job was having the right connection. The rules were clear. Wear a white dress shirt and black pants, black shoes, and be on time.

Walking in to work from the parking lot one afternoon, I was approached by a man wearing a pinstripe shirt and a dealer's vest.

"Hey, buddy, want to make a quick twenty?"

"Sure, what do I have to do?"

"I'm late for work and didn't have time to get home to get my white shirt. We can trade shirts. You can make some fast money and I won't lose my job."

I thought this was a pretty good trade, so we switched shirts. He didn't actually have the money. I would have to collect it from him at his table in the casino on my break. Unfortunately, on entering the kitchen, I'm the one who almost lost his job. In no uncertain terms, I was warned to never come to work with a pinstripe shirt or anything other than a white shirt in the future. When I ventured into the casino to collect the payment for my shirt, I realized that the dealers all had different vests than the man who took my shirt. He didn't even work there.

Another time, I was assigned the task of picking up all the room service trays deposited outside the hotel rooms. Returning with a cart full of trays and dishes, I was questioned by the kitchen manager. "Why are you back so soon? You're supposed to do the entire hotel."

"I did the entire hotel."

"Well, that's good, but you work too fast. Next time, go a little slower. We don't want anyone to lose their job."

So, this is what it takes to get along in the real world: know the right people, don't work too hard or stand out, and try not to lose your shirt in Las Vegas.

Grading pickles

For two summers in college, I worked at a local pickle factory with the job title of "Pickle Grader." This involved working outside from 6:00 PM until 6:00 AM during the cucumber harvesting season. As trucks pulled into the receiving yard, I was responsible for checking to ensure that the sizes claimed by the drivers were accurate. Cucumbers were valued based on their size. The smallest grade one cucumbers fetched more than ten times the price paid for the super-sized grade six specimens. By late night, all the pickles had been graded and we had time to kill, usually racing forklifts around the receiving yard or exploring the acre of open vats where the cucumbers were being pickled in brine.

It's amazing that I still eat pickle relish after seeing what goes on behind the scenes at a pickle factory. Cucumbers that had fallen off the conveyor belt inside the plant were routinely swept up off the floor and tossed into a vat of brine. This salty grave also became the final resting place for many unfortunate birds and other small creatures.

Years later, I discovered that my future wife was working inside the same factory at the same time that I was out in the yard, sometimes on the same shifts. She had the distinguished role of "Pickle Pounder." Her job was to fill the jars with appropriately sized cucumbers and then use a wooden mallet to make sure that each jar was filled to its capacity. Who could have known that the pickle grader and the pickle pounder would later go on to have little gherkins of their own?

What I remember most about working at the pickle factory is the opportunity to admire the sunrise from my station in the receiving yard. The rosy fingers of dawn, as Homer described it, greeted me each morning. The only problem I encountered on this job was smelling like a pickle.

Take me where the action is.

Having excelled at picking strawberries and delivering newspapers, I was ready for something more challenging. The job sounded interesting. Wanted: bookkeeper for the Airport Limousine and Taxi company. It would also have the greatest personal impact of all my work experiences.

One day, I was finishing up the books when a call came into the dispatch office. There was a fare to be picked up at the airport, but all the drivers were busy. The owner instructed me to take the limo and head out to the airport. I didn't have the necessary chauffeur's license, but the owner assured me there wouldn't be any problems.

I pulled up to the curb and found the waiting customer. A businessman, I guessed.

"Where can I take you tonight?" I enquired.

"Where the action is," he responded.

As a high school student, I had no clue where the action was. Calling in to the office was of no help. I wasn't even sure what kind of action he was referring to and the dispatcher wasn't about to give me any guidance either. Driving across town, we passed a martial arts studio.

"How about that marital arts place over there? That looks good."

Oh, I thought, *he thinks the place has something to do with marriage or women.* Now at least I knew what he was looking for.

"Sorry, I think that place is closed," I replied. I didn't want to explain that a karate experience probably wasn't what he was looking for. "I've got just the place for you."

I dropped the unsuspecting passenger off at a local tavern and instructed him to go to the far end of the bar. "Tell the bartender you're looking for some action. He'll take care of you. Upon receiving a generous tip, I immediately sped away, not wanting to find out what kind of action the rider was about to engage in that night.

It was bad enough for my conscience to be driving taxis without the right kind of driver's license. That wouldn't be my biggest concern. The owner had just purchased an ambulance which he thought would help him make some easy money. There were no EMS services in those days and no one at the cab company had medical training but that wasn't going to be a problem. He assured me that ambulance calls were routine, like cab rides only with the passenger on a stretcher, and we could drive through town with lights and sirens.

Then came an emergency call summoning us to the site of a farm accident. The owner told me to get in the ambulance. He would drive, I could take care of the patient. Pretty exciting for me until we arrived at the scene to find a teenager who had been rolled over by a tractor. *I can't believe I'm doing this*, I thought. *This kid is my age. He could die.*

His anxious family asked me if I thought that their son's spleen might be injured. I wasn't even sure where the spleen was located. Somewhere in the abdomen, wasn't it? I agreed that the injuries looked serious but reassured the family that we were going to get him to the hospital right away. The whole ride back into town, the owner seemed to enjoy the thrill of speeding through intersections while I anxiously prayed the young man would survive. Thankfully, he did. That was the end of my taxi- and ambulance-driving career.

Going through high school and college, I was a young man on a mission. My vision was set, and there would be no time to deviate from this chosen path, not even an interesting college course in which I might not succeed. By every outward measure, my college career was a success in academics, sports, extracurricular activities. I had followed the self-determination script I had crafted for my life and was a success in the eyes of others. But one area of life remained unfinished. I was alone and wanted to find the right companion to live the rest of my life with.

PART TWO

FINDING LOVE: FAITH COMES ALIVE

Chapter 6

United for Life: I'll Never Leave You

An excellent wife who can find? She is far more precious than jewels.

Proverbs 31:10 (ESV)

Therefore, a man shall leave his father and his mother, and shall hold fast to his wife and they shall become one flesh.

Genesis 2:24 (ESV)

Finding love on a street corner

I stood shivering on the street corner hoping to hitch a ride out to school one cold January morning. It was the school's intersession of my sophomore year, and I needed to get to my job in the chemistry lab. My job was to make sure the lab was properly stocked, and the experiments were set up for the students. We had lots to do and only a couple of weeks to get ready before classes started.

One car after another passed by. It looked like I would be late for work if a ride didn't come along soon. Yes! A car was slowing down, a blue Volkswagen Beetle with flower stickers on the side. Finally, a ride. Better yet, the driver was an attractive blonde whom

I presumed was a student. This was the route between the branch and main campuses of the school. With my long hair and backpack, she could see I was likely to be a student as well.

Sure enough, the driver was a freshman heading out to the main campus to pick up her books for the coming semester. We talked all the way out to school and across the campus to the bookstore where I waited as she picked up her textbooks. I didn't want our conversation to end. We talked all the way back to her car. By this time, I was late for work, but that didn't matter. I had found the woman of my life! Some people don't believe in love at first sight, but I do. On that first car ride, I knew this woman was someone special, and I was eager to get to know her better. Though I had been successful in school and work, I had never really developed any long-term dating relationships. That was about to change.

It's hard to imagine that having grown up surrounded by girls my whole life, they remained a mystery to me. My sisters were a tightly knit group, attending the same all-girls school and sharing life's secrets with each other. I don't recall them talking much about their boyfriends or school life. One time in high school, I was going to a party to meet my girlfriend. As I walked in the front door, she made her exit through the back door with another guy. Crushing. Then there was the girl who chased me around the pool table trying to get me to kiss her. She was eventually successful.

A couple of weeks after the best hitchhiking ride ever, classes resumed. Walking with a friend into my Psychology 201 class, I paused in amazement. The only seats available were right in front of the girl with the blue Beetle! The teacher told us to turn around and introduce ourselves to somebody in the class. I think I was facing her before he had even finished giving those instructions. After class, I invited her to join me for a cup of coffee. Standing in line in the school cafeteria, I asked her how she wanted her coffee. She said she'd have it with cream and sugar, the same way I did. Little did we realize that neither of us had ever drank coffee before that day. I'd just thought it sounded mature to get together for coffee.

From that point on, we talked each day after class, and I eventually summoned up the nerve to ask her out to the annual Snow Ball which would be taking place in a few weeks. I still remember pacing back and forth in the kitchen of the home I was sharing with a friend, picking up the phone, then putting it down again, heart pounding. Several friends and I had gone out for dinner to an all-you-can-eat pizza buffet where we consumed one hundred pieces of pizza between us (we kept track). Whether the pizza helped strengthen my courage for the phone call or not, I couldn't say. With my stomach churning, I dialed her number and asked her out.

"Oh, thanks for asking," she replied, "but I don't think I have anything to wear."

Rejection. Was this her way of politely turning me down? I had used that line myself once before to avoid going out with a girl I barely knew.

Not ready to give up so easily, I countered, "I'm sure you can find something. How about if I call back tomorrow to see?"

I didn't realize that right after our call, Diane drove to a fabric store, picked out a pattern and the material and started sewing. Within a week, she would have the dress completed.

When we talked the next day, she said she had found an outfit that would work for the dance. My anxious request for a date was accepted! When I shared my good fortune with my roommate, he told me his parents were friends with the girl's family and assured me he could give me directions to her house.

Following Brad's directions, I arrived at her house a few weeks later with a flower and a small box of chocolates. I had seen this done in the movies, and it seemed like the right thing to do for one's first date. Wait a minute, who is this answering the door? A puzzled man wanted to know what I was doing disturbing his evening. I was at the wrong house, and worse for me, he didn't know where the girl lived. In the days before cell phones, finding the right address involved driving around until I could locate a payphone so I could call and get directions. That was Valentine's Day, 50 years ago, and Diane and I have been together ever since.

The dance was held at the Northland Hotel in downtown Green Bay. I liked the Northland. It was a Green Bay landmark where my family had occasionally gone for breakfast to enjoy their signature dish, Schroeder Eggs (scrambled eggs with tomatoes). The second-floor ballroom was decorated in a winter theme. How appropriate for a young couple who had met on a street corner on a cold winter day.

We talked about our backgrounds, interests, and the jobs we had held and discovered we had something in common. We had both worked at the local pickle factory. We agreed to see each other again at school, though I insisted that we meet in the library where I could keep up with my pre-med studies.

It would be an understatement to say that I was always considered a good student, most comfortable in the classroom and library. Schoolwork never had to deal with any competition other than part-time jobs until I met Diane. By her own admission, she was not exactly headed for the Dean's List. Our study habits were radically different; something had to give. After we met, I would invite her to study with me at the library. Sitting across from her, I would be poring over my textbooks, taking notes, and completing assignments when I would feel this tapping on my foot. Interrupting my studies, I would look up to see if there was something she needed. "Is it time yet for a cup of coffee?" More than once, I responded to the effect that we had only been studying for ten minutes or so. The coffee would have to wait.

How my future mother-in-law saved the day

Love at first sight doesn't mean there weren't challenges along the way. Our first crisis came when we attended a reception at the Chancellor's home. The evening started with a lecture presented by a distinguished guest speaker, a highly regarded author. Diane and I sat back in the last row of the auditorium, where no one would be watching us, not entirely focused on the program. As young people in love are prone to do, we were occupied in conversation about other matters. My attention was divided as I tried to hear enough of the talk to make some intelligent comment at the reception, should that be needed.

After the lecture, we were invited to the Chancellor's house along with several other representative students. Our school was getting a reputation for some of its innovative classes, and the Chancellor wanted to show off some of his prized students.

At the reception, the esteemed guest asked Diane a question about her coursework. I wondered if he had noticed us in the back row. Was this his payback for our lack of attention to his important lecture?

"And who are you?" he questioned the frightened-looking student with his aloof tone.

"And who are you?" Diane jokingly replied, not recognizing him as the evening's speaker.

"Tell me about your coursework," he pressed her, circling his prey, blood in the water, closing in for the kill. Thankfully, he didn't ask what she thought of his talk.

Silence. Diane froze, unable to give him any answer at all! I tried to cover for her by offering some comment about how we sat too far back to see him clearly.

But the harm had been done and nothing I said helped the tense situation. After that embarrassing moment, we escaped outside to talk and face the hard reality. These types of social situations were going to inevitably come up if I pursued my career in medicine. I resolved to be vigilant for potential times like this in the future and was confident we could work this out. She wasn't so sure and didn't want to talk to me anymore about it. It appeared that we might break up over this event. She didn't want to see me again and suggested I go on with my pre-med program without her. She didn't think she would ever fit into these types of gatherings and more of them lay in our future.

The next few days were unbearable but I wasn't willing to give up on the dream of a future life together. I wanted to tell Diane that she was more important than the advancement that came from such gatherings. It was a long and lonely ten miles from my apartment on campus to Diane's home across town. I'd never walked that far in my life and had plenty of time to rehearse my words. Diane's mother answered the door. She liked me and refused to go along with Diane's unwillingness to see me. I can still hear her summoning Diane to come right up from her basement bedroom so we could talk. I guess it's always good to be on the right side of your girlfriend's mother when times like this arise. We got engaged shortly thereafter.

Most of my visits to Diane's house were after school and on the weekends and didn't see her dad very often. I wondered what kept him away so much. Then I realized he worked long hours in a local paper mill to support his family. He was the first shift worker I had ever met and his work schedule didn't always line up with my visits. Over time, Lloyd taught me how to throw horseshoes and play dart ball, but mostly, he taught me what it meant to be a faithful husband and father. Diane and I played board games with her family, attended church, and shared many meals and other activities, the kinds of things an intact family does. This became the model for the family life I hoped to have when we had our own children.

Another major problem to be confronted was that we were from different religions, Catholic and Protestant, oil and water. It took a long time for our families to accept that goodness could be found in persons from other faiths. After our engagement came the challenge of designing a wedding service consistent with the religious beliefs of both families. We were married in Diane's church but had my parish priest involved as well. This way, our marriage would be acceptable in our parents' eyes.

The wedding almost didn't happen thanks to my indiscretion the afternoon of our rehearsal. The prior day, Diane was trying to demonstrate her new golf swing to her mother and accidentally hit her in the nose with a golf club. Just what every mother of the bride hopes for, a bloody nose and a black eye, and a trip to the Emergency Room for stitches.

Then a more serious threat arose. I had gone golfing with my brothers and members of the wedding party, and we stopped for a hamburger and a beer before heading over to the church. One pitcher of beer led to another and pretty soon, I had to go directly to the church without the benefit of a shower or a shave. We stopped at a drug store and picked up a disposable razor, so I could shave in the car but without the benefit of any shaving cream. I wasn't a pretty sight on arrival at the church and Diane almost walked away from the rehearsal.Worse than my appearance was my failure to appreciate that drinking put the whole wedding in peril. I still had a lot to learn.

Newlyweds start their life journey

Our honeymoon set the tone for the first several years of our married life, when we never had enough time or money to have a real vacation. With only a couple of hundred dollars and two weeks before starting medical school, we drove all the way out to California and back in eleven days. We stopped in Las Vegas to see my brother Joe and his wife Sally, then headed up to Davis, California where my dad was doing an anesthesia residency, another stop on his personal quest to find the right job for him and his new family. En route, we spent a night north of Los Angeles at Pea Soup Anderson's, where we enjoyed their signature menu offering, an unlimited amount of pea soup, followed by the only motel stay of our honeymoon. Neither of us anticipated the impact several bowls of pea soup would have on our intestinal tracts. For me, this brought back memories of a similar experience in the backyard tent. It was the most memorable night we would ever spend in a motel even if not the most romantic. For the rest of the trip, we camped along the way, even spending one night in Joe and Sally's front yard after our late-night arrival at their Las Vegas trailer home.

As young married students, we were determined to keep our expenses under tight control so we could remain debt-free. At the time, we could only afford one new pair of jeans per year. For entertainment, we watched movies on campus or got together with friends. Our one-bedroom apartment was cozy, some would say intimate, furnished with distress sale furniture like our flood-damaged mattress and assorted hand-me-downs. The focal point of our living room was a desk–a secondhand door placed onto two file cabinets. The hole for the doorknob was perfect for the power cord for the table lamp. Bookcases were made of boards and bricks. We didn't have much, but we were in love, so that didn't matter. We rarely ate out and, for a while, had to walk the one to two miles to school or the grocery store after our car was totaled in an accident.

Priorities

Married life can be difficult for anyone, even those who aren't involved in rigorous programs of study. Medical training was going to be my path to the life I dreamed of. I was well prepared for the academics, but nothing prepared me for the challenges medicine presented to our marriage.

It was the night before a major biochemistry exam, and I felt nervous and unprepared. Many of my classmates had studied the subject in college but I hadn't. I wanted to study more for the test, but Diane wanted to talk about the stress of being newly married and in medical school. We never seemed to get around to talking about her dreams of school, career and family. *Couldn't this wait*, I thought. This was a big exam and if I failed, I might flunk out of medical school. What to do? Study more for the exam or take the time to meet my wife's needs? She wanted to have a career too, but mostly, she wanted my attention and presence in her life.

My decision to take time to meet Diane's needs helped define the way we would communicate throughout our marriage. The biochem exam would have to take care of itself. I wondered if my parents had faced similar dilemmas and how they resolved them. I suspect medicine won out more often than not. I don't recall the grade from that exam; it doesn't matter now. One failed test wouldn't have flunked me out of medical school. I passed the biochemistry test at school and the more important test at home. Another step in becoming the kind of husband I wanted to be. I must have done alright on that and my other exams to have been chosen for the Alpha Omega Alpha Honor Medical Society.

Together, we had successfully established the kind of marriage we wanted to have and how we would resolve the inevitable conflicts of married life. Growing up, I had been trained to run away from conflict, a common feature in children of alcoholics. Not being confrontational by nature, I tended to submerge my emotions hoping to avoid negative interactions whenever possible. This may have been possible when single, but it would be a recipe for disaster in a marriage. In this case, the teachings of the Bible were life-changing. While we might get angry or disagree from time to time, we agreed to never allow ourselves to go to bed without acknowledging the issue. If we were unable to resolve a disagreement late in the night, we would try to do so the following morning. We were determined to establish the best home we could, following the best advice available. I was going to avoid the path my parents had taken and rewrite the script of my family life with a more favorable ending.

The following years would be marked by my ongoing studies and Diane's efforts to find her own path through school and work. After the first semester of medical school, she put college on hold for a year to work at a bank. The demands of medical school were just too much for both of us to be pursuing our dreams at the same time. Our energy went into getting our marriage established before starting our family. We enjoyed traveling together, pursuing outdoor activities and hobbies like photography, and overcame the initial threats to our relationship. This early commitment to our marriage would sustain us through the challenges to come. We were also confident our background and education would help make us good parents as well.

Chapter 7

A Family of My Own

These commandments that I give you today are to be on your hearts. Impress them on your children. Talk about them when you sit at home and when you walk along the road, when you lie down and when you get up.

Deuteronomy 6:6- 7 (NIV)

After 7 years of marriage, it was time for us to start our family. We both loved the idea of having several children though not as many as my parents. Was waiting to start a family the best way? Should we have started sooner? We'll never know but the delay gave us time to get our marriage on a solid footing. We could enjoy each other's company while I completed my training before taking on the responsibilities of raising children. I just assumed we were ready to be parents as long as we followed the guidelines of the experts. We had both grown up in large families, and, with my pediatric training, I'd have all the answers to any questions about bringing up our children. If only that were true as illustrated by the following incident.

The ultrasound

The confident pediatric resident and his wife looked at the ultrasound screen with amazement. "There's our baby: heart beating, fingers and toes perfectly formed." I had just studied ultrasound and wanted to demonstrate my newfound skills of interpretation. "See this? It's our baby's head!" I proclaimed with self-assurance. "Well, actually, that's the buttocks," interjected the amused technician. "The head is over on the other side." So much for trying to impress my wife.

Something similar had happened previously when we were picking cherries in an orchard north of Salt Lake City. Diane wanted to pick from one tree but deferred the decision to me, given my prior experience working in a cherry orchard. When the owner walked by, I solicited his affirmation of what an exemplary tree I had selected. "Actually," he replied, "that's one of the worst trees here. We planned to cut it down but didn't get around to it before the season started." Lesson for me: Listen to your wife!

Diane and I trained for the Salt Lake Marathon in the second year of my residency. We wanted to accomplish that 26.2-mile race before bringing a newborn into the household. The race was held on Pioneer Day, July 24th, and the temperature was over one hundred degrees by the time we entered the downtown area for the finish line. Diane had been coughing some before the race and later found that she actually had pneumonia. Nevertheless, we both finished the race and, for me, it was the start of many decades of recreational running.

Our first pregnancy was pretty uneventful apart from concerns that Diane wasn't gaining weight as expected. She had resumed her running and physical fitness training even though pregnant. The doctors were concerned that our baby wasn't growing well either. In reality, Diane's exercise program was keeping her weight down.

The following spring, I was on call the day Diane went into labor. She was out shopping with one of our residency friends when her water broke. She quickly came up to the hospital and waited for me in the call room until I could arrange for coverage. We headed off to Holy Cross Hospital where twenty-four hours of labor ensued. The main thing I remember about the labor was that when I tried to follow the Lamaze guidelines by rubbing Diane's back, she angrily ordered me to keep my hands off of her! With all the stress of thinking we might have an underweight baby, we were happy to deliver a 8 lb. 5 oz. little girl.

The doctor as a dad

We wanted to prove our naysaying friends and family wrong about the impact of children on our lives. Having children wasn't going to change our style of living. How wrong we were. There were times one of us would sit outside on the front porch while the other tried to comfort our inconsolable new baby. None of my reading could guide me on this. Another time, I was determined to take Rachel cross-country skiing and fashioned a sled that could be attached to my waist with a belt adapted from a backpack. The contraption looked great on paper. After securing Rachel into this make-shift sled, we started out on the trail but within a few feet, her sled hit a root, tipping her over head-first into a snowbank. So much for the brilliant idea of cross-country skiing with a baby on a sled. On an airplane trip, we spent much of the time rinsing diapers and actually draping them to dry over the seat. So much for the notion that babies don't change your life.

We celebrated Rachel's first birthday much like any family with cake smeared all over her and anyone else within her reach. A few months later, Diane began to question why she had so much trouble losing the weight she had gained during her first pregnancy. She had taken quite a liking to M&Ms and I insightfully commented that perhaps the one-pound bags of M&Ms weren't helping her weight loss efforts. (I must have missed the class on being a sensitive husband.)

Once the tears subsided, Diane told me about the queasy feeling in her stomach. I asked her to lie down on our bed and performed an abdominal exam. Her uterus was almost to the level of her navel meaning she was likely about 4 months pregnant! I brought in a urine sample to the hospital and came home with a smile and a rose. Diane immediately broke down in tears on learning that she would soon have two children only nineteen months apart. Tony was born five months later and Sam two years after that.

Having grown up in a medical family, I was familiar with the doctor taking care of their own family. Having a doctor for a dad can be a good thing but there are certain drawbacks. One morning when I was in grade school, I entered the dining room in my bathrobe as Dad was eating his breakfast.

"I think I should stay home from school today. My throat is a little sore."

"Go out to my car and bring me my medical bag."

"Actually, I think my throat is feeling better. I'll just get ready for school"

"Let's take a look just to be sure."

Why did I ever say I had a sore throat? I immediately regretted ever making any comments about staying home. Following a brief exam in the dining room, Dad reached into his bag and pulled out a syringe full of penicillin.

"Down with your pants." In went the needle. "Good!" Dad exclaimed, "We caught this in time. Now you can get off to school." I trusted his judgment and never doubted he had my best interests in mind.

Some kids might at least get to stay home from school after getting such a shot, but not in our household. All day I sat carefully at my desk, squirming on one cheek, the other sticking out into the aisle. I never missed a day of school or work after that for years. My dad's approach to treating family carried over to how I looked after our own children as seen in several incidents.

Tony had developed a sore throat for which he was hospitalized overnight for observation. During my training, I had seen many children with epiglottitis, a potentially fatal swelling of the throat. An anxious night ensued as I slept next to Tony's crib repeatedly checking his breathing and monitoring his condition. Health issues take a completely different look when it's your own child.

After that time, I tried to resist following my dad's example until the day Sam needed stitches after falling and hitting his head on a bookcase at the library. Diane brought him to the clinic where I persuaded a surgeon to repair the gash between his eyes. I didn't think the stitches looked all that good, but I wasn't a surgeon.

Diane and the kids went home and within a couple of hours, Sam had climbed up onto the kitchen table and fell once again, pulling out all the stitches. I was too embarrassed to call the surgeon to repeat his work, so I sutured Sam myself. I took pride in my suturing ability having practiced extensively by making counted cross-stitch Christmas ornaments on twenty-two stitch-per-inch hardanger fabric.

Strapped into the papoose board, Sam cried, "Daddy, Daddy" as I numbed up the area and placed a new set of stitches. Maybe it's just my imagination, but the outside scar from those stitches is virtually indistinguishable now that Sam's an adult. I'm afraid I don't know what inside scars might have been inflicted in my efforts to take care of things myself to save face.

Rachel, Tony, and Sam were born within a span of three and one-half years. Diane and I were outnumbered and had enough to keep us fully occupied. We didn't believe in the idea of intentionally spacing our children, so it was four years later when we had Emily. She was a delightful child, sociable and agreeable, and one who readily made friends in our neighborhood. One time, when we were living in Salt Lake City, Diane and Emily came to pick me up from a talk I had given at a local hospital. Emily had gotten a handful of markers and was unusually quiet all the way to the hospital. When they arrived, a friend met them and commented that Emily looked purple. Diane replied that yes, Emily was quite verbal only to realize that the friend was referring to Emily's new hair color.

We completed our family with Peter, the baby from the convent. We had moved back to Green Bay following my two years of allergy practice in Salt Lake City and settled into the convent adjacent to the Christian school where Diane was going to be teaching. This was the former Catholic girls' high school my sisters had attended. The nuns' rooms had been converted into small apartments for use by people affiliated with the school. Less than a year later, Peter was born. Arriving six years after Emily, he received more of our attention than any of our other kids. I still cherish a photo published in the local newspaper of Peter, age four, and me cross country skiing at the Reforestation Camp.

Involved parents

We considered ourselves to be involved parents, always looking for ways to contribute to our kids' lives, from volunteering at their schools to helping with homework, science fair projects, and Pinewood Derby cars. Having played soccer in college, I was able to coach youth soccer even during my allergy fellowship, primarily because none of the other parents had any soccer experience. Maybe they didn't have the time. That is, except for one parent whose daughter was the star of our team. This dad would constantly yell at his daughter throughout the game exhorting her to run harder, pass better, shoot more effectively. That wasn't going to be my style but maybe I could have pushed my own kids to strive for excellence.

We tried to establish family traditions beginning with Bible reading and Advent programs, board games, camping, field trips and vacations. We wanted to build a sense of unity and bonding within our home. The most enduring of these activities was our annual pilgrimage to the strawberry patch where I wanted to instill my love of fieldwork into our children. But they never needed to labor in a strawberry patch all morning to earn a couple of dollars per week. Motivation is everything. In reality, those trips to the strawberry patch did more for me than for our children. For me, they became one touchstone of stability when our family life later came under strain. For the kids, the trips were more a matter of eating strawberries. That is, when they weren't tipping over my flat of berries or complaining about the amount of time we spent out in the hot sun. Nobody complained, however, when we got home and made strawberry freezer jam to sustain us for the coming winter.

The family on vacation

Part of my script for family life included scenes of childhood vacations, even if they didn't always turn out as intended. I recalled how my parents had taken my brothers and me on a trip to Washington DC, and I wanted to give our children this type of memory as well. I probably should have thought that there might be some troubles on vacation like the time my brother Johnny got his head stuck in a revolving door at the hotel or when the family drove off without him from a gas station. I planned to do better when I became a parent.

For Diane and me, family vacations were always a great challenge but none more so than the time we went to Disneyland. Walking around the massive park, we suddenly realized that Tony was missing. We frantically searched for him only to have him show up mysteriously an eternity later, seemingly out of nowhere. He had walked up a ramp onto an overhead tram and rode around the park, wondering why we were all running around. "What were we looking for?" he later asked us. "Didn't you see me waving at you?"

One of the high points of our family vacation experience was a train trip from Salt Lake City to San Francisco. We arrived at the station a little after midnight and were scheduled to leave a couple of hours later. There were two trains on the same track, and we were instructed to get ourselves onto the train on the left side. Once we were comfortably settled in our seats, the conductor said we would be making it to Las Vegas in so many hours and then on to Bakersfield California. I realized there was no way we were on the right train as neither of those cities was on the way to San Francisco. We had mistakenly gotten onto the wrong train!

The conductor radioed the dispatch office and found that the San Francisco train had already departed but was then delayed by some type of electrical problem as it was leaving the train yard. We grabbed our stuff and raced along the railroad tracks, kids in hand, Emily on my shoulders. Breathless, we made it onto the right train and left for San Francisco shortly thereafter. I could envision our family looking like some characters in a movie. Who are those people scrambling to catch the last train out of town in the middle of the night? What are they running toward? Or away from?

As we arrived in San Francisco, the Chinese New Year's parade was going right in front of the station. We stayed at the Presidio, a former military outpost converted to a hostel and enjoyed many of the sites of San Francisco, most notably Fisherman's Wharf where we took a ferry to Alcatraz. On board, a man was talking to a group of students. I asked their teacher if we could join their group and she said yes. The speaker was actually a former Alcatraz inmate! He presented a firsthand account of life in that infamous prison, and later I purchased a copy of his book as a souvenir of our experience. Back at Fisherman's Wharf, we gorged ourselves on a Ghirardelli Chocolate Earthquake Sundae and later consoled each other that our ensuing stomach aches were worth it for the pleasure of devouring this massive creation.

We didn't need to go away on a vacation to have memorable family experiences. When Diane and the kids persuaded me we needed a pet, we found one that seemed right for our family at the animal shelter. We couldn't have been more mistaken. Within a couple of days of her arrival in the home, the animal started growling at the kids and even bit Emily on the cheek. We tried to return the dog to the shelter but were told we'd have to wait until they reopened the following Monday.

Diane and I had dinner plans with some friends, so we carefully instructed the babysitter and the kids to keep the dog penned up. Midway through our dinner, I called home to check with the babysitter to see how things were going. She replied something to the effect that the police had just left our house, the Fire Department team was still interviewing neighbors, and the Animal Control people insisted on a phone call the following morning. Nice joke, I thought. Except it wasn't.

If only the kids had listened to our instructions. As one opened the kitchen door, another opened the front door creating a critical alignment of opportunity for the penned-up dog. Out the front door she raced, chased by our kids and the babysitter. In itself, this might not have been so bad, but the jail break occurred at the worst possible moment. Our neighbor was getting out of her car, having just been discharged from the hospital where she had been treated for a nervous breakdown. She must have been shocked to see this strange animal racing right toward her and her screaming children.

Quite a commotion ensued as parents, children and a babysitter all chased after the frightened dog. The neighbors reported the problem to the 911 operator and before long, our quiet circle looked more like a crime scene, crowded with the police, Fire Department, Animal Control officers and curious onlookers. The dog was impounded and later found to have some type of brain problem, explaining its erratic behavior.

Getting away to attend a professional meeting posed challenges of its own. On one occasion, Diane's parents came out to watch the kids while we went to a medical meeting for several days. They and the kids reportedly had a good time in our absence, and we were able to relax knowing that our children were in good hands. On our return, we drove up the circle to our home to find grandparents standing on the front porch waving happily. I imagined they were pleased that their more structured approach to childcare had kept the children safe in our absence. The children were also waving, proudly standing on the roof over the front porch!

Smarter doesn't mean wiser

To an outside observer, our family appeared to be thriving, but serious cracks had already begun to show. Like my own parents, Diane and I couldn't agree on how to approach the kids' behaviors. Diane shared this with our pediatrician who offered to refer us to a counselor. I resisted his advice thinking my professional training gave me some special insight into parenting and school problems. Perhaps it did for other people's kids, but I had a blind spot when it came to my own children. Being right and looking good in front of others was more important to me than being together in the way we raised our family. Overriding Diane's judgment was one of my biggest failings. Sadly, this wasn't the only time. Training and education may have made me smarter, but certainly not always wiser..

Sometimes, our family paid the price for my mistaken priorities. Once, when Emily was in middle school, she and I had the opportunity to attend a father-daughter weekend at Lake Lundgren Bible Camp. I was teaching Adult Sunday School at our church at the time and felt I couldn't leave my class unattended. The other dads in the class, including several church leaders, were at the retreat with their daughters. Family life was a higher priority for them. In letting Emily down on that occasion, I was following in my dad's footsteps, putting my own interests and needs before hers.

My father used his work to avoid the pressures of home life. I didn't recognize that over involvement in spiritual pursuits was just as bad, and with the same ultimate effect. It took a long time for me to forgive myself for this episode and even longer to learn from these kinds of mistakes. Some people can be slow learners where it matters most.

So that's my own family, five children born in three different cities, interspersed in five moves, two training programs and four medical practices. A dizzying odyssey from Madison to Salt Lake City to Chanute Air Force Base to Green Bay, to Madison, Salt Lake City and back to Green Bay. Somehow, Diane oversaw all these changes and managed our household while I listened to the siren call of career and personal dreams.

While there are many positive memories of these early years with our family, some of my own shortcomings were becoming apparent. I didn't recognize the impact of repeated moves on Diane and our children. When we lived on the Air Force base, surrounded by close friends, we flourished until it came time to move. Without the supportive structure of the military, we tried to establish ourselves in the community, but never felt like we fit in the private practice world. Driven by my fear of failure and need to look good, I couldn't see my family objectively and admit when one of us needed help. After all, I was a well-trained pediatrician who was supposed to have all the answers. At least for everyone else. How could my own kids have behavioral or emotional problems that required professional evaluation? This question was going to be an ongoing issue in our family.

When we moved to Green Bay from the Air Force, our family life settled down for about three years. We lived across the street from a city park where we enjoyed the swimming pool almost every summer day. Diane's Mom came over to spend some time with us, but we never really felt like there was any great enthusiasm from the grandparents for getting involved with our family. They already had work and other responsibilities to attend to. The same could be said about our siblings who had lived in Green Bay much of their whole lives, each with networks of friends and relationships we never quite found a way to break into.

Chapter 8

Finding God: A New Life of Faith Begins

Therefore, if anyone is in Christ, he is a new creation. The old is gone, the new is here!

2 Corinthians 5:17 (ESV)

Even if my father and mother abandon me, the Lord will hold me close.

Psalm 27:10 (NLT)

My childhood observance of religion changed when I moved out of the house for college. No one could force me to go to church anymore; my spiritual life was up to me. I didn't really question what I had been taught in religion classes, it just didn't matter as much to me. In college, I had approached religion like many others of my generation: someday important but not quite so soon. I didn't realize that this approach has been common for a long time. St. Augustine reportedly once prayed, "Lord save me, but not yet."

Faith and religion

Growing up, I was fairly religious: altar boy as a youth, parish council as a teen, Mass on Sundays, always following the rules. Church was important but it certainly didn't dominate my day-to-day life. Like many Catholics, I comfortably picked and chose which rules to follow among the Ten Commandments and the many Church teachings.

Things began to change when I met Diane. Her family was Protestant; I had never met any non-Catholics before. They took spiritual matters seriously like mine did, but with a much greater emphasis on the teachings of the Bible. They attended a liberal Christian Church where the pastor gave thought provoking sermons that included a Bible verse or two before discussing material from *Psychology Today* and classical literature. Their faith was built into family traditions in a way I had never experienced apart from attending Mass or saying the rosary. Labor Day weekend meant a trek to Lake Lundgren Bible Camp in northern Wisconsin, the same camp where Diane's grandmother had volunteered decades earlier. Now I was being grafted into their annual tradition, joining a new family in more ways than one.

Over a weekend of Bible teaching and traditional Christian hymns, we enjoyed games, sports, and other family-oriented activities. This was the first place I heard the Christian gospel spoken with passion and clarity. The camp speakers had an amazing ability to take a short passage of Scripture and expound on it in detail over a series of five related messages, all leading to a strong call to action. This was all new to me and left me with many questions: What was this teaching about being born again? How can they say I don't have to work my way into heaven? Does God really care about me personally?

In medical school, Diane and I occasionally went to Mass but usually found it more interesting to take the weekend off for bike rides, camping, and getting together with friends. My medical school downplayed the importance of spirituality and religion. For students, the teaching was emphatic: a good physician never lets personal beliefs impact the way they approach patients. Religion should be kept in a separate private realm of thinking.

Moving to Salt Lake City, the home of the Church of Jesus Christ of Latter-Day Saints (the Mormons), changed our religious perspective. We were now surrounded by people who took their religion seriously. Some of our Mormon neighbors began to show interest in becoming friends, inviting us to use their washer and dryer. Discussions about religion became common when we got together with them until we realized that this newfound friendship was prescribed by their church as a way of converting their gentile neighbors. When we told them we weren't interested in joining their church, the laundry service closed down. Our relationship wasn't based on us at all. We were just a mission to be accomplished.

With the pending birth of our first child, we had to get more serious about spiritual matters and started attending church more regularly, even after nights on call. I slept through many sermons those days. I wanted to support Diane by going to church with her and began to develop a sense that something was missing in my life in the spiritual realm. We had to decide what we were going to do about religion, since we came from different backgrounds. Diane resolved that concern by agreeing to convert to Catholicism. Our baby would be baptized in the Catholic Church. We took a class at the Newman Center at the University of Utah campus to get up to speed on the teachings of the Catholic Church. For me, this refresher course in the church I grew up in started my own spiritual awakening. Starting a family changed me before our first child was even born.

The religion class was intended for Diane, but actually had a greater effect on me. One of the talks involved a priest teaching about the Psalms. The words of Psalm 136 still echo in my head. Each verse of this Psalm said something about God but ended with the same refrain - *O give thanks to the Lord for he is good; For his loving kindness endures forever.* I had never appreciated the beauty of the Psalms before.

Who could have imagined that the words of Scripture could be so lyrical, so beautiful? I soon found myself drawn to reading short Bible devotionals on my own. My concept of God was changing from the all-powerful and far-off scorekeeper to an all-loving nearby Savior. Unlike my own father, God the heavenly Father wouldn't change his mind about loving me and leave me behind for some other pursuit.

Something else was happening to me that I had never expected. We began to talk with friends about faith-related issues. By the time Rachel was baptized, I had been given my first personal Bible, a Catholic version with a picture of the Pope in the front. I started a lifelong habit of reading it regularly.

While many Catholics are content to have been baptized as an infant, Evangelical Christians will often speak of being "born again," through which they personally accept the role of Jesus Christ in their lives. Some believers experience a dramatic life-changing conversion, akin to St. Paul who experienced Christ on the road to Damascus. Most others, myself included, come to faith in Christ in a far less remarkable way. For me, the moment of final acceptance of God's lordship of my life came on Ash Wednesday 1982. In accordance with my Catholic upbringing, I had been fasting all day. Diane had taken Rachel and Tony up to Green Bay to visit her parents, so I was home alone. After work that evening, hungry, reading my Bible and praying for direction, I had a sudden sense that the time had come for me to make a decision. I fell to my knees and submitted my life to Christ, no longer able to live on the sidelines of faith. From this point on, I would be all in.

My first Bible study.

I was a changed person from that point on! Faith in God was going to be the thing that tied all of life together. Having just made this new spiritual commitment, I felt it was time for me to get more serious about reading the Bible. What better way than to study it with others? The following Friday at the Air Force bowling league, I recruited members for something I had never done before.

Pins crashing, beers and sodas in the cupholders, the cheering bowlers were focussed on strikes and spares. Some had come to the Friday night bowling league at the base lanes with their specially drilled bowling balls and custom wrist braces, intent on pursuing that elusive perfect 300 game. For most of the rest of us, the evening was a social outing, the scores a sidelight to the conversations and refreshments. Diane and I were new on base, and this was the best option to get out of the house for an evening.

I walked up and down the lanes, waiting to talk to people between frames.

"Hey, want to start a Bible study?"

"Sure. Sounds like a good idea. What will we study? Who will lead it?"

In a flurry of spiritual fervor, I recruited friends and neighbors from among the fellow bowlers to join me in a Bible study. Moving to the Air Force base, I was now surrounded by committed Christians both at the hospital and in our neighborhood. While surprised by my newfound enthusiasm, my new group agreed to join me in a study of the Book of James.

The only problem with organizing the Bible study was that no one seemed inclined to lead it. Undeterred, I took that upon myself, even though I had no personal background in reading the Bible, much less leading a home Bible study. In taking on this responsibility, I learned something that would guide me for years to come: once a person makes a commitment to serve God, needed abilities will follow. God doesn't call the equipped, He equips those He calls. Bowling for Jesus!

At the time, Diane and I were leading the folk choir at Saturday night Mass on base even though I was only able to play four chords on the guitar. Skill and talent were optional requirements for service. Our son Tony sat in his infant seat as we led the worship music and is now an accomplished guitarist with my Yamaha guitar from those Air Force days one of his preferred musical instruments. I must humbly accept some credit for the great example I provided in those early, formative years. We also taught a baptism class for expecting parents.

While active at the Catholic chapel, we also started attending First Baptist Church just outside the base on Sunday mornings. We had visited there once at the invitation of some friends. When we returned for another visit about a year later, the pastor surprised us when he remembered our names and a couple from the church invited our family (all five of us) to Sunday lunch at their home. They explained how they regularly prepared a full lunch meal for whomever they would happen to meet that particular Sunday. Where does one find hospitality like this?

This church also had a Bible teaching program for adults. I had never experienced anything like this in my life as a Catholic where only priests and specially trained people were considered qualified to teach the Bible to others. So we went to church twice every weekend, but were we Catholic or Protestant or some combination of both? We longed for a spiritual identity.

While struggling with this dual citizenship, I began to understand that faith was actually about a relationship with God not a religion with lots of rules. This new understanding found its ways into our baptism class. All was going well until a visiting priest sat in on the class. He was shocked and considered us to be heretics, definitely better suited for a Protestant church. (We can be thankful that burning heretics at the stake has fallen out of practice.) Our role in teaching the class was summarily terminated. Worse, we were deemed unfit to serve as proxy godparents for our friends' child. In response, we quit the guitar choir, left the Catholic chapel, and worshiped at the Baptist Church for the remainder of our Air Force tour.

Our spiritual identity question was settled when we moved back to Madison for my allergy fellowship. Upon visiting an Evangelical Free Church in our neighborhood, Diane ran into one of her college friends who invited us to come back the following Sunday. After attending there for several weeks, I volunteered to help out in the Sunday school class for four-year-olds. I figured my level of Bible understanding probably matched theirs so we would be a good fit.

Bible teacher

I fell in love with teaching Sunday school through that experience and wanted to help others learn to teach as well. On a couple of different occasions, I would recruit a hesitant friend to join me in teaching children. One of them went on to be ordained as a pastor.

A central teaching of evangelical Christianity is that the Bible is God's true and inspired word and is the foundation for our understanding of God and his ways. I approached the Bible as if it were one of my textbooks, highlighting, making notes and checking off the chapters. Several years after my conversion experience, I read about a famous Christian preacher who began reading through the Bible every year at the age of eight, a practice he continued for over sixty years. How could I do any less than an eight-year-old child? From that point on, I was determined to read through the Bible yearly, usually in fifteen to twenty minute blocks of time each morning. To learn more about the Bible, Diane and I both became involved in Bible Study Fellowship, a rigorous Scripture study program that has had a lasting impact on us both. Later, our pastor taught me how to teach the Bible to small groups. With his encouragement, I started teaching adults and even studied Biblical Greek to become a more effective teacher.

Just like when I tried to answer all the questions in fourth grade, I was quick to share what I was learning with others. So why should this be any different when what I was learning was the Bible? Unlike prior generations, many people today aren't very knowledgeable about the Scriptures (some would even say they are "Biblically illiterate"). They are only vaguely familiar with its beauty and richness, unaware of the frequent references to Biblical themes in our daily lives. I saw it as my personal mission to rectify that situation.

On one occasion, we spent a year in Adult Sunday school going through the message of the entire Bible. This was a particularly ambitious effort that required a study of systematic theology. Of course, I had to learn this myself and considered taking seminary-level classes. Each week, preparation for Sunday school involved hours of late-night study to develop a lesson plan based on the inductive study method of Aristotle (i.e., drawing conclusions from the study of particular details of Scripture).

In addition to reading the Bible, memorizing key Scripture passages can change one's life. I first learned of this practice through Diane's parents when they made a concerted effort to memorize Bible verses in their sixties. Diane's Dad carefully typed out the verses so he and Diane's mom could quiz each other. He became quite interested in how many pages of Bible verses he had accumulated, as if getting this down on paper was the main point. One day, as he was showing off his hard work, Diane's mom commented, "Lloyd, why don't we just memorize more and type less?"

One way to keep Scripture in mind involves writing out a passage each day on an index card which is then carried throughout the day. I first learned this practice while my brother Luke and I attended Bible study for professional men. The leader of our group had invited a prominent business executive to meet with our group. The guest shared how after completing his morning Bible reading, he would often write a Scripture verse on an index card. He would then place the card on his desk to be seen by the countless visitors to his executive office. He shared how, on many occasions, this simple index card prompted spiritual conversations. I adopted this practice for myself. The index cards transformed my approach to sharing the Bible with others, regardless of the church they attended or their spiritual beliefs. Since our guest speaker later became ordained as a deacon in the Catholic Church, I could assure people that daily Bible reading wasn't only for evangelical Christians.

I became known for always having a Bible verse handy at work and I looked for appropriate opportunities to share one. On occasion, something would come up in the course of a patient visit related to the Scripture passage I had read earlier that very morning. Was this a coincidence or was it something else? With the index card in my pocket, I was in a position to share this. When the recipient was a patient, I asked their permission before sharing Scripture with them. My offer was rarely declined.

Writing out a Bible verse many days a week for many years is one way to get a large collection of index cards. Our kids still tease me about this habit. One Christmas, Sam gave me 1,000 index cards for a Christmas present. I think I've used them all over the years. As a child, I had collected baseball cards and traded them with my brother's or friends. As an adult, I've moved on to sharing cards with more enduring value.

From all the teaching came opportunities to preach at our church. Some of the individual messages included "*Nehemiah, my brother, the Servant Leader,* and *Catch the Wave.*" I delivered a spiritual message at my sister Margaret's wedding and another one at our high school class reunion.

Given my traditional Catholic upbringing, it was inevitable that there would be some conflict with my mother's Catholic beliefs. One day, as we were talking about spiritual matters, she asked, "Where did I go wrong with you and your brother Luke?"

"Well, Mom," I replied, "if by going wrong you mean that Luke and I love our wives, are devoted to our families, and try to live our lives according to God's Word, maybe it would have been best if you had "gone wrong" with all of the kids." That was the last time we talked about my evangelical Christian beliefs.

Despite our differences, Mom and I respected each other's beliefs and we continued to talk about the Bible regularly. Over time, she also began reading Scripture daily. Thinking back, I can see that the way I handled mom's question was not the most sensitive approach. It just reminds me of how much grace my mother extended to me and how she fully accepted my new beliefs. When mom passed away, my family chose me to deliver the eulogy. I based my message on her favorite passage of scripture, "Count it all joy my brothers when confronted with trials of every sort." (James 1:2)

Problems at church

For me, faith is based on a personal relationship with God and is meant to be lived out in a community of fellow believers. This meant we needed to find a new church with every move. On returning to Green Bay to start my allergy practice, we attended the newly formed Evangelical Free Church where we became friends with the pastor and his wife. I was able to serve as an elder and Bible teacher and we felt as though we really belonged. Troubles came when I tried to apply my critical thinking background from medicine to issues at the church. As an elder at the church, we had to consider purchasing property and building a new church facility. I had questions about the wisdom of this move. To the pastor, even asking questions about such matters was considered a sign of disloyalty. I was thoroughly reproved and began to wonder if we were in the right church.

Our relationship with the church worsened when Diane and I tried to donate use of our commercial property. Our church had planned to establish a downtown ministry and we had extra space in just the right location. The church started using the space for outreach to the area and began to see some fruit from that effort. Then a foreign mission opportunity came along, and the church leaders abruptly lost interest in reaching out to our own community. We felt betrayed and never fully trusted our church leaders from that time on.

Growing up as a Catholic, it had never occurred to me that we would look around to worship at different churches. Catholics typically stayed with their home parish until the bishop assigned a new priest to lead them. Evangelical Christians tend to shop around until they find a church that best meets their needs, spiritual consumers. Unfortunately, people who leave a church often bring their hurts and problems with them. The cautionary saying has been noted that if you actually do find the perfect church, please don't join it because it won't be perfect anymore.

People leave evangelical Christian churches for any number of reasons. Our pastor eventually resigned under pressure from the congregation over his style of leadership. Although we had our differences, he always supported adult Bible education. His successor had a different perspective and canceled my adult education class. This was a sad day for me. I had devoted many years of my life to teaching the Bible helping many people grow in their faith and their understanding of God's Word. Now that was taken away along with my sense of purpose in the church. Some in my position would have fought this change, but I didn't. I couldn't fight this battle and still be able to worship in that church. My sense of loyalty to this church had finally reached its limit; It was time to leave, time for another move. Sunday morning was for worship, not drama. Thankfully, we've been able to find a new church to attend without any angst or drama, only worship, with an opportunity to discuss the Bible in small groups.

Whether my experiences with individual churches have been good or bad, there is no question that my relationship with God has been at the center of my life over the last 40 years. People may disappoint, reject, and even abandon us but God promises He never will.

Reflecting back, I wonder if all this time spent on Bible study and teaching took too much time away from my family. Was I avoiding the more important responsibilities I had toward them? Or was it more that daily Scripture was my lifeline in the midst of turbulent surroundings in my home and workplace? In any case, in the Bible I had finally found that God's Word answered my questions about life's purpose and meaning and held my life together.

PHOTOS

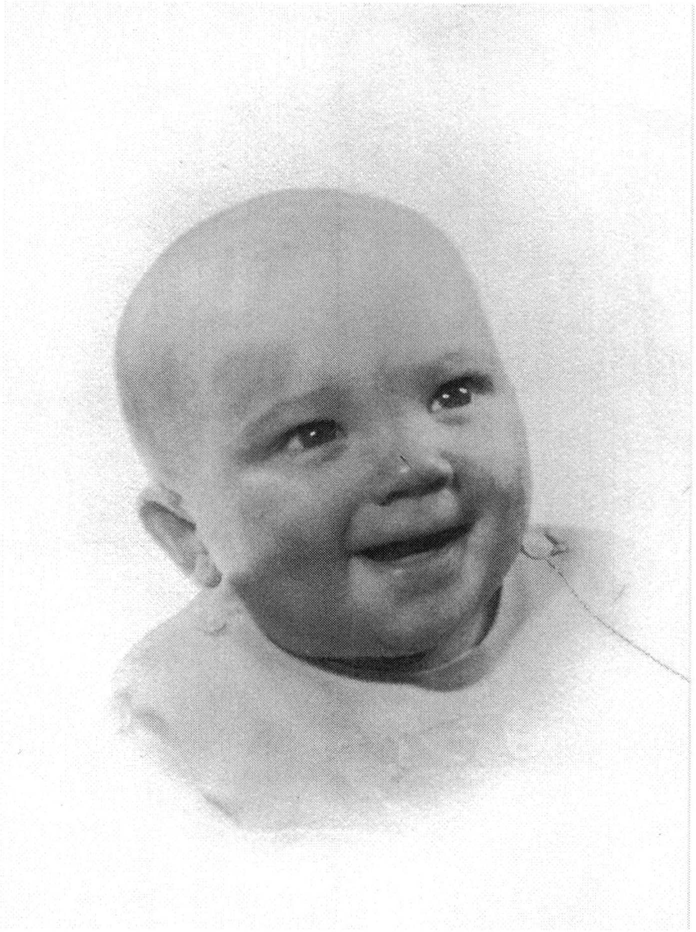

Age one

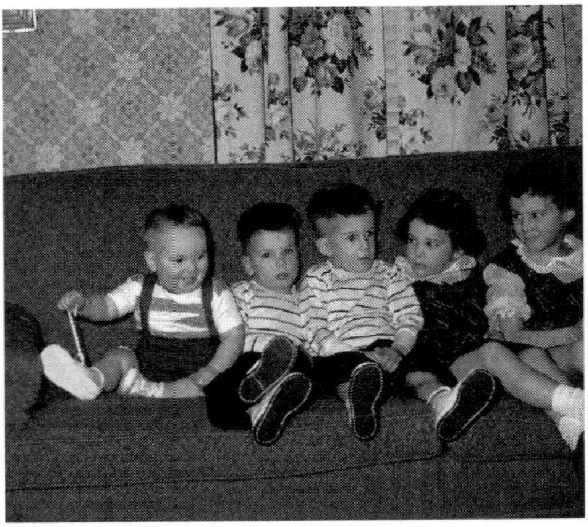

South Dakota—Jim, Joe, Mark, Susie, Kathy

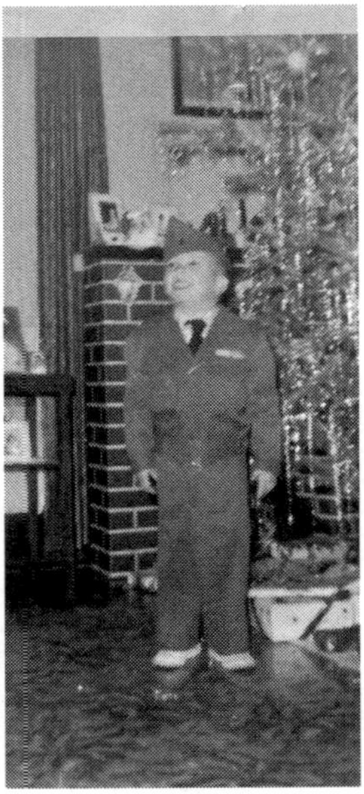

Junior Officer

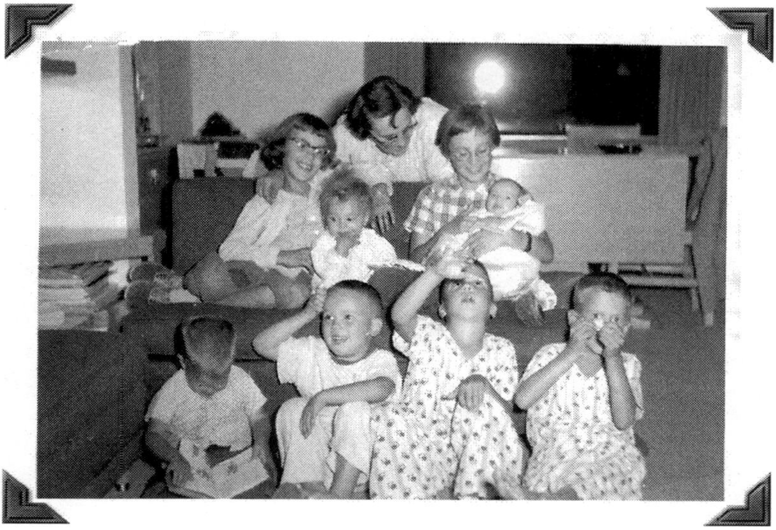

Bedtime

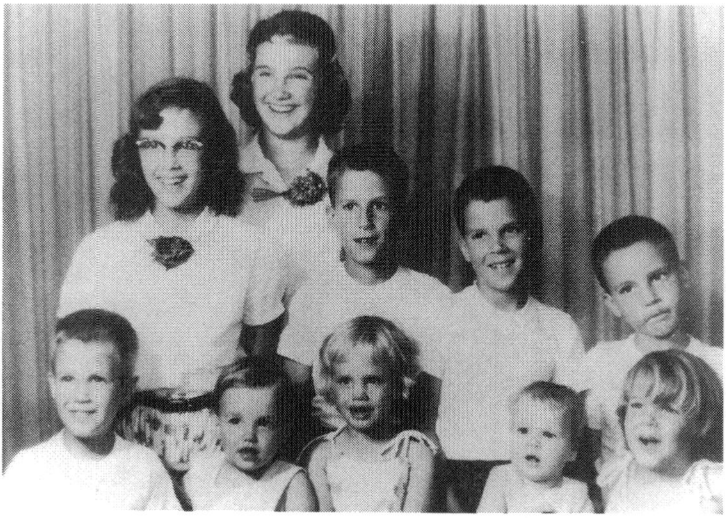

My signature pose

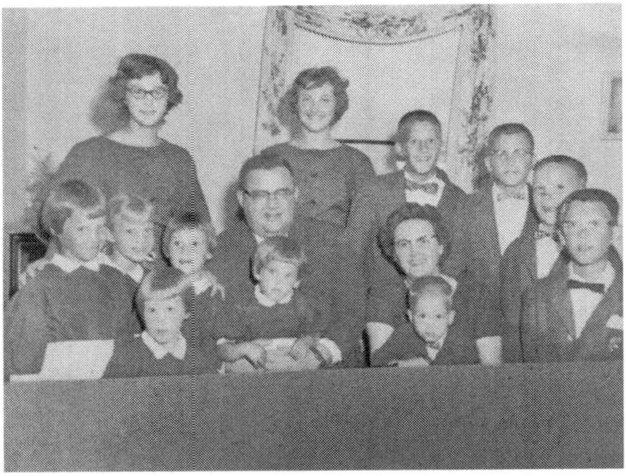

Family with Lucy on the way

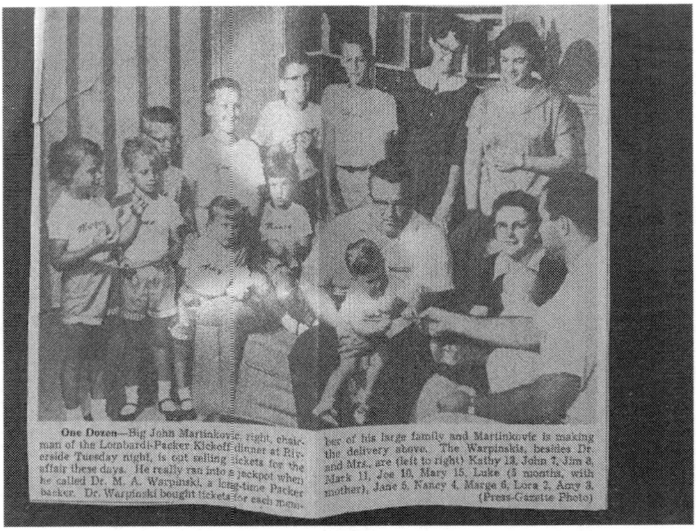

One Dozen—Big John Martinkovic, right, chairman of the Lombardi-Packer Kickoff dinner at Riverside Tuesday night, is out selling tickets for the affair these days. He really ran into a jackpot when he called Dr. M. A. Warpinski, a long-time Packer backer. Dr. Warpinski bought tickets for each member of his large family and Martinkovic is making the delivery above. The Warpinskis, besides Dr and Mrs., are (left to right) Kathy 13, John 7, Jim 8, Mark 11, Joe 10, Mary 15, Luke (3 months, with mother), Jane 5, Nancy 4, Marge 6, Lora 2, Amy 3. (Press-Gazette Photo)

Packer tickets

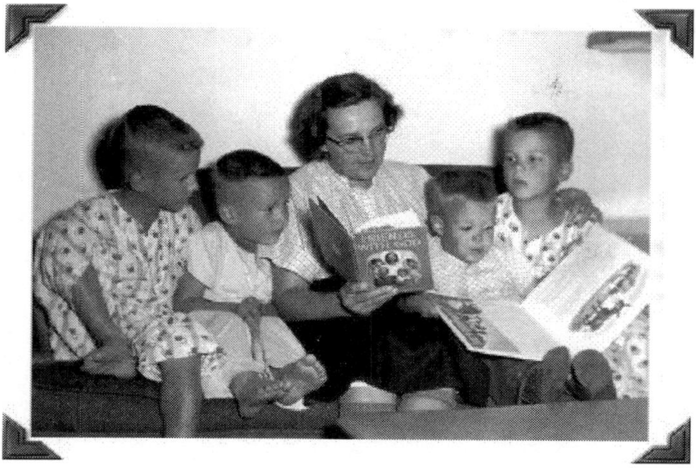

Mom and the Four Boys

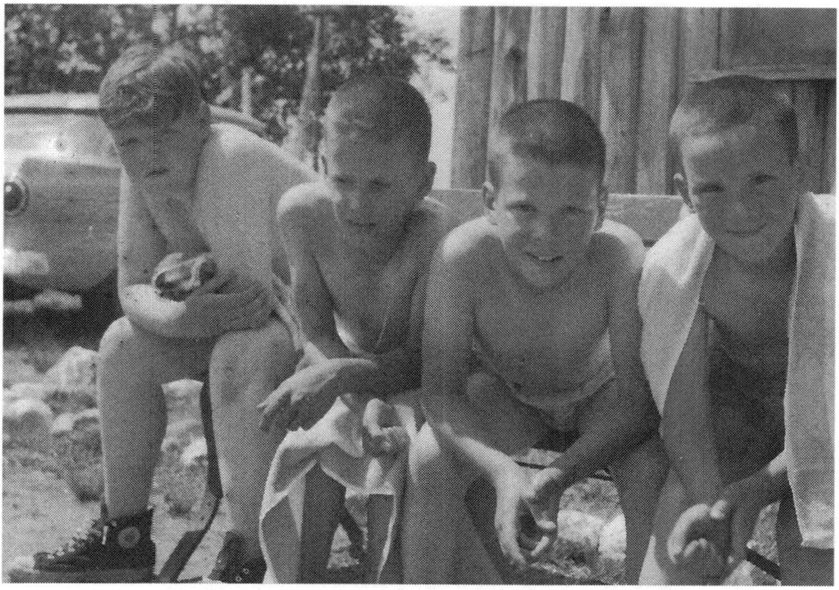

At summer camp with Mark and Joe

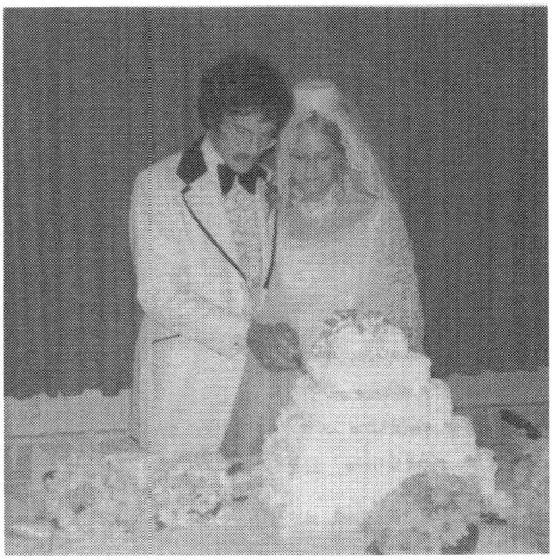

Wedding Day

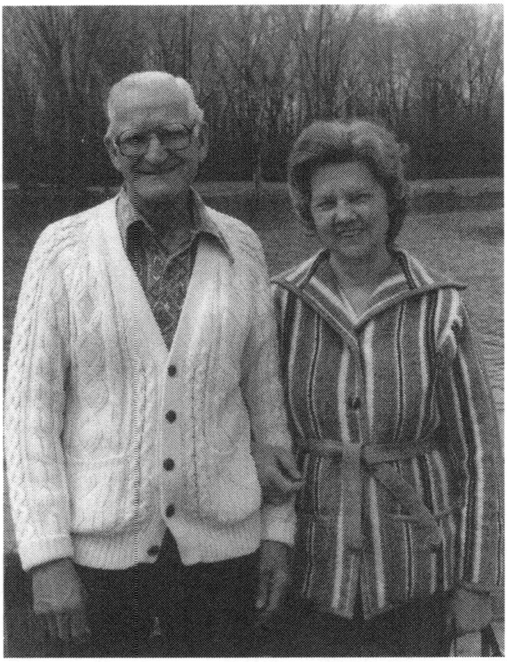

Diane's Parents—Lloyd and Mary Lou

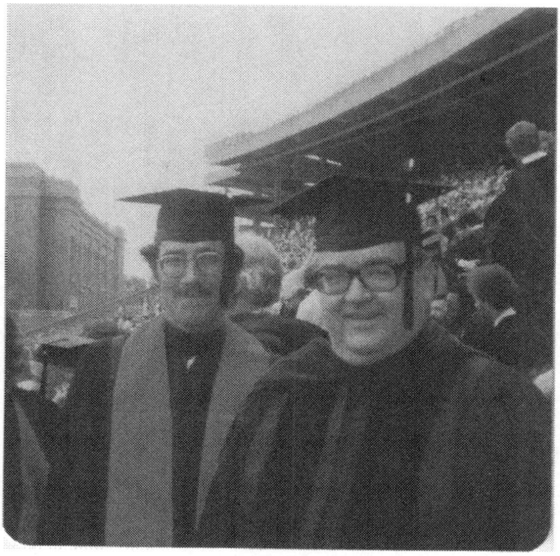

Medical school graduation

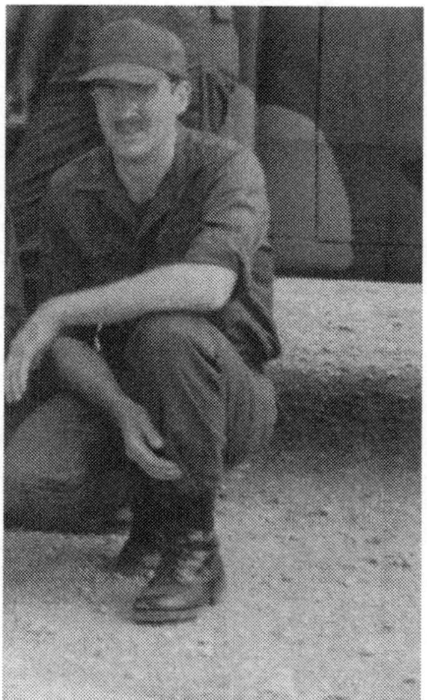

Air Force days

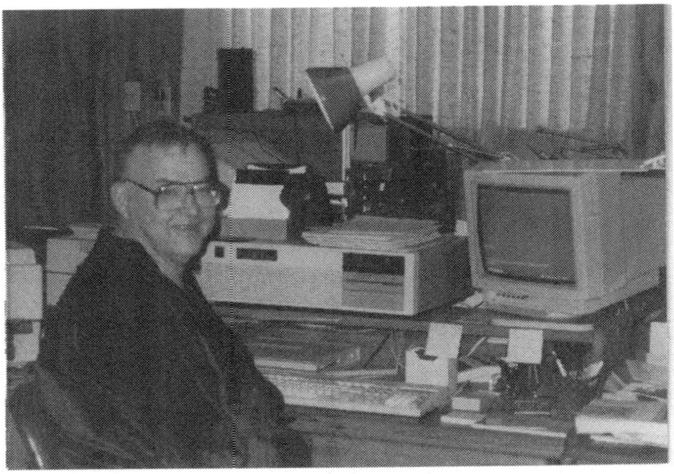

Dad at computer

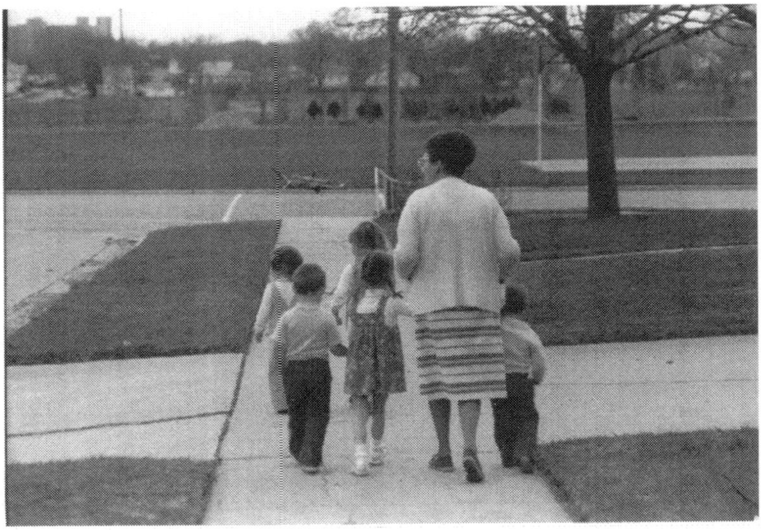

Mom and grandkids walking to the park

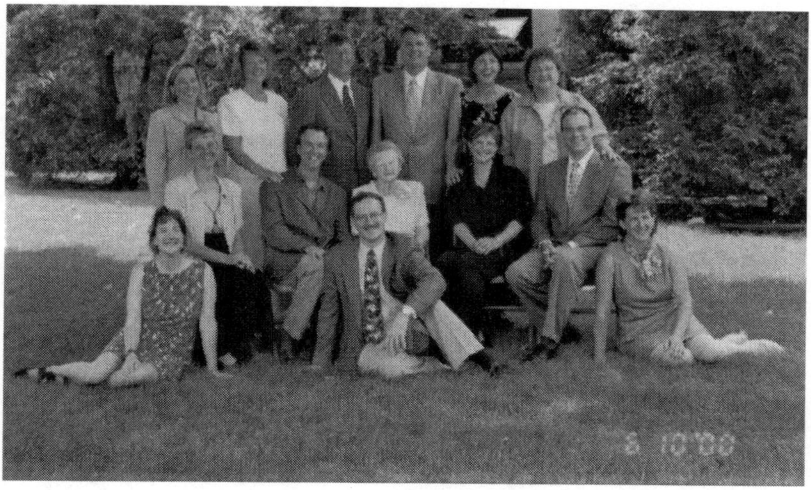

Mom's 80th Birthday

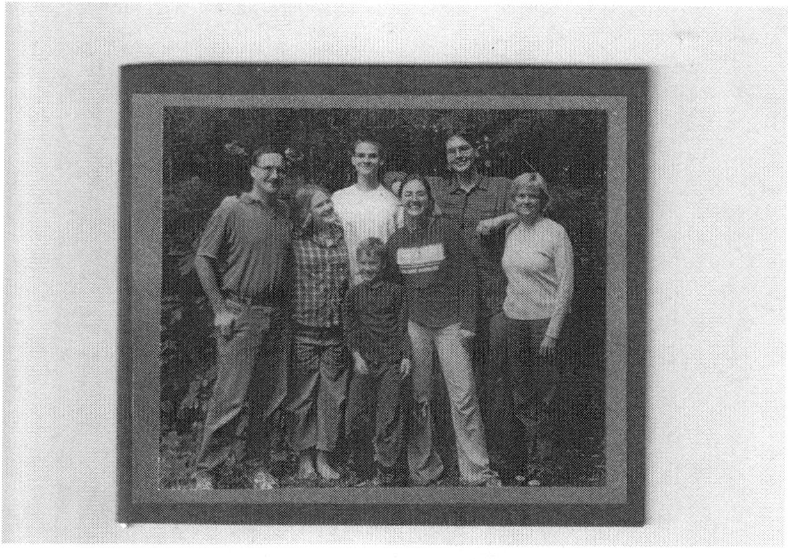

Family at Bible Camp

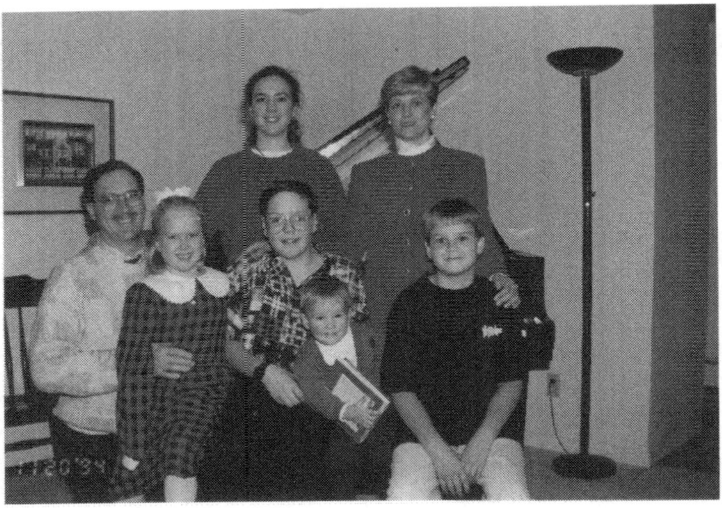

Family Christmas

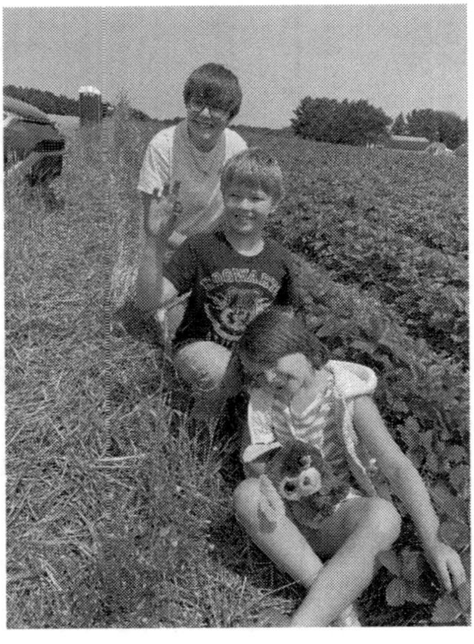

Picking strawberries with grandchildren

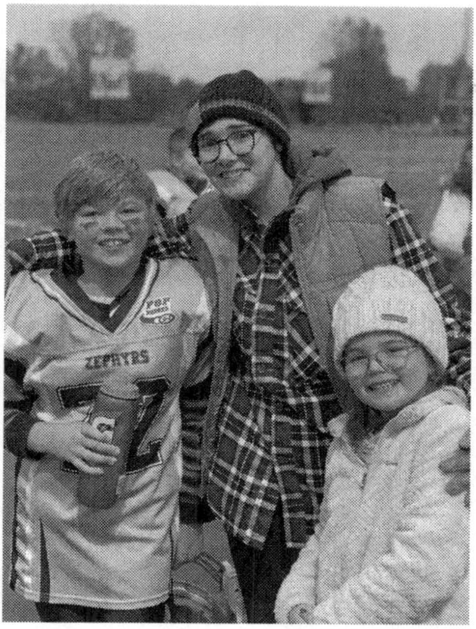

Grandkids

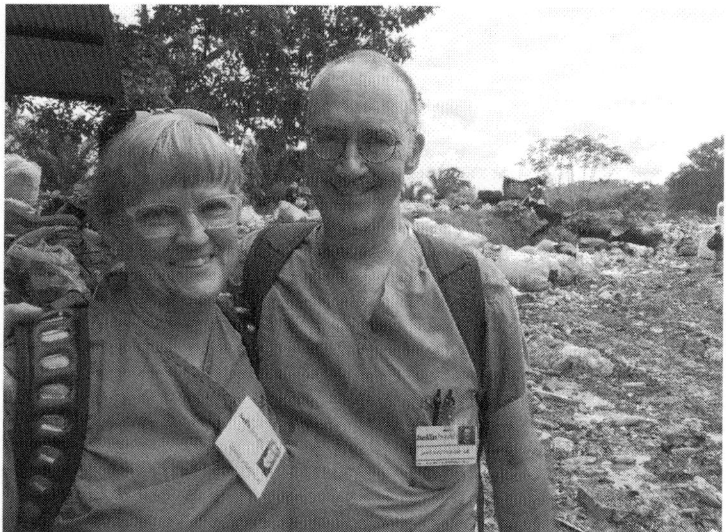

On the mission field in Guatemala

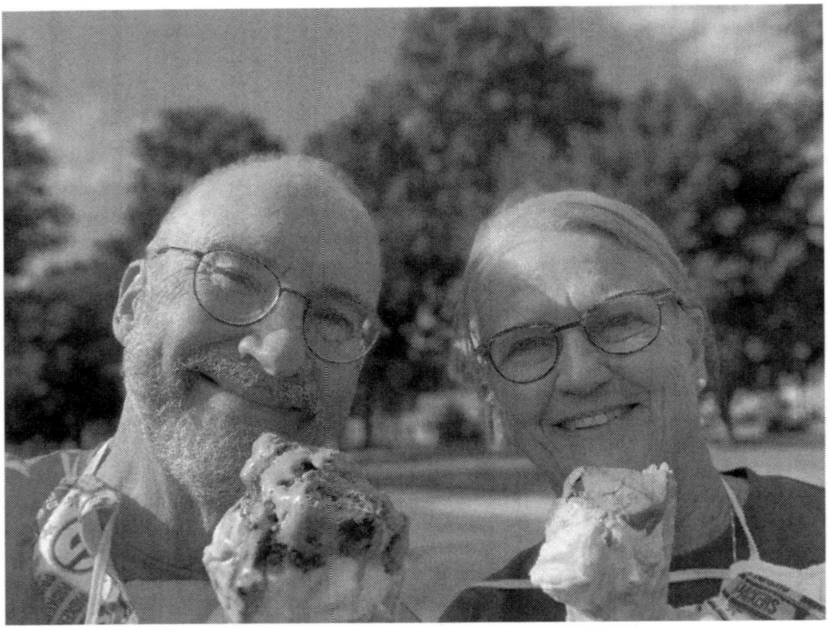

Retired life

PART THREE

MEDICINE: PUTTING FAITH INTO PRACTICE

Chapter 9

Becoming a Doctor

He who began a good work in you will bring it to completion.

Philippians 1: 6 (ESV)

On rounds with Dad

Growing up in a medical family and spending time around hospitals showed me advantages medicine provided for the doctor. Sometimes, Dad would take several of us kids along on house calls while he would run in to see a patient. In theory, this was to be a quick visit while the kids were to remain patiently in the car. In reality, he would return up to an hour later. What could be taking so long? Dad was a large man, generally weighing over 300 pounds, maybe in part because his appreciative patients often provided a light lunch after the doctor visit was completed.

At other times, several of us kids joined Dad when he ran a few errands before making rounds at St. Vincent Hospital. As was the routine, he instructed us to remain in the car until he returned. We had other ideas like sneaking into the doctor's lounge for snacks, having elevator races or playing hide and seek in the hospital basement where we avoided getting too close to the room with the sign "Morgue." On one occasion, Joe and I took a pair of Dad's pants just retrieved from the dry cleaners. We each got into one leg and managed to fasten the pants around our chests and then walked around the hospital, greeting patients and hospital staff.

I recall attending a Packer game with Dad in the dark ages before cell phones and pagers. In those days, a doctor would notify his answering service of his whereabouts when on call. And Dad seemed to be on call a lot. It seemed like during every game, the public address system would call out, "Paging doctor number such and such, paging doctor such and such, call the hospital immediately." I never understood why they didn't just call the doctor by name, but thought the doctor they were trying to reach must be really important for 60,000 fans to hear them summoned.

I was relieved it wasn't doctor 369, my dad. He was frequently called away from family activities for urgent problems. But not during this game. We could relax and enjoy the rest of the game together. Years later, they would be calling my number when I got to be a doctor.

Whether sitting in the back seat of the car, playing in the hospital or cheering at a Packer game, our family was always aware that Dad was a doctor. I wanted to be one too.

Medical School

My thoughts about becoming a doctor started sometime around fourth grade. But why? Was it my experience with reading from the medical book with my dad, making the house calls or seeing the respect doctors had, I couldn't say. I admired my dad and his work, and entered medical school right out of college. I never thought of any other option.

Medical school started the day after we returned from our honeymoon. We lived at Eagle Heights, the married student housing at the University of Wisconsin. Getting to school several miles away was accomplished by walking, taking a bus, or riding my bicycle. We couldn't afford a parking pass on campus. The curriculum was standard for that era with two years of basic sciences followed by two years of clinical training.

Much has been written about the life of medical students dissecting a cadaver in the anatomy lab, enduring endless lectures, and studying countless hours. For me, being a student was a little more involved. I had a job from grade school on so it seemed natural that I would work evenings at the medical school library to keep us from having to incur any debt. Diane tells me I smelled like formaldehyde for the whole first year when we were learning gross anatomy. I wasn't sure if this was an upgrade from smelling like a pickle, but at least the odor came with the prospects of better times ahead.

Physical diagnosis class followed gross anatomy and opened up the mystery of the human body in a way I could never have imagined. For the first time, I would be learning to examine a living person. This involved mastering the techniques of physical examination including the use of specialized instruments like the stethoscope for listening to the heart and lungs. The examination of the ears required use of a tuning fork. When hearing loss was identified, the response to the vibrating tuning fork could help determine its cause. As with other exam skills, we first practiced on ourselves before attempting the technique on others. Imagine my shock when I could hear the vibrations of the tuning fork in my deaf ear! The "permanent" hearing loss I'd grown up with had been misdiagnosed.

Here I was, a medical student correcting the work of a trained specialist! My professor was excited to have a person with a real physical finding for the group of students to practice on. And practice they did. First they reproduced my findings and then went further to see if the nerve to my ear was working properly. This involved squirting ice cold water into my ear to see if my eyes would start to dance. (For the medically interested, this is a test of the balance center in the inner ear.) That wasn't enough to convince the professor who then had the students spin me around in a special chair. More dancing eyes.

All the tests turned out to be for my benefit. Since I didn't have any money to pay for expensive ear surgery, the ear specialist performed the surgery as a professional courtesy. Perhaps he was also compensating me for being the class guinea pig.

The ear surgery involved replacing a portion of a bone in my middle ear that had never properly developed. I was fully awake throughout the entire procedure so I could tell the surgeon when the middle ear bones were properly reconnected. The change in hearing was instantaneous. I could hear everything, including conversations in the hallway outside the operating room. When we returned home from the hospital, I could hear car doors being closed in the parking lots outside our apartment. What an amazing thought that our hearing is actually that sensitive. Within a few days, I no longer heard all of those extra noises. My brain filtered them out so I could pay attention to things of greater importance.

The day I became a "real doctor"

Throughout the world, there are rituals through which people gain entry into a group. They might involve some physical trial like surviving in the wilderness under harsh conditions, maybe even killing a wild animal. All requiring some type of transitional experience. The clinical years ushered in greater degrees of responsibility which over time help the student form a new identity as a physician. Medicine has its own rites of passage, its own gauntlet of experiences that make one feel like a member of the profession.

For some students, seeing yourself as a doctor starts with getting accepted into medical school. New school—new you! But the classes are just harder, and the hours longer.

For others, it's the white coat ceremony. New coat—new you! But the white coat is simply something worn on top of regular clothing.

Still others might wait until they walk off the stage with the letters MD after their name. New degree—new you. But titles don't change a person.

My rite of passage was different. It changed the way I viewed myself, no longer the student in a white coat posing as a doctor. And more importantly, it gave me a foretaste of what that was going to mean for me..

It wasn't detecting the cause of a hearing loss not found by the specialist.

It wasn't starting an IV that had eluded the intern.

It wasn't finding the pneumothorax missed by the radiologist.

I had done all of those, but they weren't what made me feel like a real doctor.

It was my first night on call, a third-year medical student assigned to the psychiatry floor at the university hospital. At the end of the day of rounds, lectures, and workups, I was entrusted with my first pager, like the ones the residents and attending physicians carried. I was instructed to contact the hospital immediately should I receive a page.

It's hard to describe the excitement and the sense of responsibility of being on call for the first time. I was a student doctor, the one at the end of the line on rounds, the one nobody missed if you weren't there.

Now, for the first time in my career, I might be needed to perform some valuable service at the hospital. Any moment, my pager could go off and I would be summoned. Perhaps my medical history and physical exam might help unlock the mysteries of some patient's diagnosis.

My wife and I decided to celebrate this big event by going out to dinner, a rare treat in those days of tuna casseroles and hamburger helper. We chose a nearby fast-food restaurant, close enough should an emergency arise.

We were just sitting down to eat when it happened.

My pager went off! The moment I was waiting for. The moment I was going to be needed, a full-fledged member of the team. I rushed over to a payphone to call in. Diane started to gather up our food.

My pager went off again! It must be something really important. What's taking so long for them to answer?

Then the unit clerk picked up.

"Hi. This is the third-year medical student on call. You paged me." I expected an urgent call for me to rush back to the hospital.

"I'm sorry, are you sure about that? Nobody here is looking for you. You should check your pager."

My pager went off a third time! This time I noticed a restaurant worker turn off a timer before depositing a batch of French fries onto a tray. The paging stopped.

I've had countless days and nights on call since then, and sometimes, I really was needed for emergencies. But most of the time, my pager remained a silent reminder of the life I had chosen.

Now, even when not on call, I find myself checking my right hip, like reaching for a phantom limb sending its errant signals, calling me to be prepared.

The time comes when getting paged is no longer special. It's something you learn to live with, the rite of passage you've made to enter the profession of medicine.

But none of that could have been on my mind the night I first saw myself as a real doctor, even though I was only paged by a French fry machine.

Medical school was a transformative experience in other ways. The medical student never graduates as the same person who enrolled four years earlier. For me, there were many experiences that permanently changed me and altered my perspective on life, leaving indelible impressions decades later. I can still recall some of the individual patients from the medical school days. Mr. N suffered greatly from the bone pain of metastatic prostate cancer. Each day's rounds involved trying to find some way to get him relief but without the adequate tools that are now available. There was Mr. S, the man at the Veterans Hospital with early-onset dementia in the room with the Dutch door. Each day we would walk by on rounds, he would ask us, "Hey, buddy, can you just open this door and let me out of this room?" One day, he was found walking down the railroad tracks behind the hospital. I wondered who had opened his door.

In the psychiatry unit, a young woman suddenly developed bloody urine while in the hospital. Her urinalysis revealed a broken pencil lead, not the anticipated kidney stone. I had never known people to hurt themselves like that. Why did she do it? On the Pediatric floor, we cared for many children with cystic fibrosis at a time when the condition was uniformly fatal before adulthood. I can still picture one particular patient, beautiful, red-haired teenage girl, full of life and energy. I had taken a personal interest in this girl with advanced cystic fibrosis hoping she would be the exception to the grim survival statistics. Then one night when I was off duty, she started bleeding into her lungs and never recovered. She was the first patient I lost.

To get more experience, students were dispersed across the state for their clinical training. I was assigned to the Howard Young Medical Center in northern Wisconsin. Driving there with Diane, I paused our conversation to envision what was before us: new place, new people, new responsibilities. As we shared our concerns, we knew that we had to literally cross that hill if we were ever going to achieve my goal of becoming a doctor. My preceptor was a surgeon who allowed me to assist in surgery, develop my suturing skills, and experience life as a community physician. Mostly, this was a good experience, though there was the time that he took me out to his property where porcupines were destroying his pine trees. He told me it was his prerogative to deal with the animals as he saw fit. I only recall shooting a porcupine out of a tree with a pistol. How I hit it I couldn't say. We'd had more than enough to drink by this time. I woke up to try the porcupine meat for dinner. I think it was tough. At least that's what they told me.

That night of drinking scared me. I found the alcohol too enjoyable, and had to face the fact that I came from a family of alcoholics. I had toyed with drinking before, like the time we'd hidden the bottle of Southern Comfort at my grandma's house. I was going to be a doctor, and I wouldn't let alcohol or any substance ruin my career. More than that, alcohol had contributed to the breakup of my family. I couldn't let that happen to my marriage. I was beginning to change as a person as I took on my new identity as a physician. After that night in the northwoods, I would keep a strict limit on drinking.

Patient care experiences also started to change my view of myself as a capable doctor. A young woman came to the emergency room complaining of the acute onset of breathing difficulties and chest pain. Otherwise, she seemed perfectly healthy. She had not injured herself nor was there any other explanation for her problems. Physical exam didn't give any clues as to the cause of her troubles and her chest X-Ray was reported to be normal. Something didn't seem right, so I took a closer look at the X-Ray for myself and found that a tiny amount of air had leaked from her lungs into the chest cavity. Back to Radiology I went, film in hand to have my finding confirmed by the radiologist.

For the first time in my career, I found an abnormality on X-Ray that hadn't been detected by the specialist. I was becoming capable of making a diagnosis on my own. The young woman had developed a spontaneous pneumothorax, a leaking of air into the chest cavity. With the correct diagnosis, we were able to provide the care she needed. My confidence soared.

Not all experiences in medicine turned out to be so positive. For me, competition in the field of medicine began early. Good grades in high school paved the way for acceptance to the right college where pre-med students competed for admission to medical school.

Next came competition in medical school itself, starting with getting good grades in the basic science courses, followed by opportunities to get clinical experience, and, finally, for securing a spot in a desirable residency. This was quite frustrating for me, as I'm not the pushiest person and would often find myself shunted to the back of the line whether in the patient's room or the operating room. As a result, I could never get close enough to a laboring woman to deliver her baby. My reluctance to speak up for myself was starting to impact my medical career. I had to find a way to compensate for this.

Getting clinical experience was necessary to make a favorable impression on the faculty, especially the ones writing letters of reference for residency applications. My strategy was to envision myself as being fully dedicated to whatever service I was rotating through as if that were going to be my career pursuit. This served me quite well in surgery where I read the entire textbook over the course of the rotation. I repeated this course approach to studying medicine and pediatrics, each with their own thick text, each to be methodically read as I checked off chapters in the table of contents, a master "to-do" list. When a student shows this level of interest, the faculty naturally offer them more experiences.

There was a drawback to this type of inner pressure to perform. One night, a young girl came to the children's hospital with a problem she had kept hidden from her parents for many months. It turned out to be a cancerous growth in her upper thigh near her groin and she was too embarrassed to tell anyone. I stayed late to do a complete workup but then had to ride my bike home in the dark. While my patient workup was complimented as being done well, the same couldn't be said for my bike ride home. Gliding through an unlit intersection, I was struck by another bicycle and suffered a concussion. Sadly, my bicycle didn't do as well as I did in recovering from the accident. The other rider and her bike fared better. I learned that trying to be a conscientious doctor comes with a cost.

Medical school could be humiliating at times and not just for the students. At a teaching hospital, patients are cared for by a large team ranging from the most experienced physician to the lowliest student. On one occasion, the surgery team was making hospital rounds with the Department Chairman. As we proceeded from room to room, the attending physician or a resident would present the case to the Chairman. Probing questions would follow, ostensibly designed to teach us important points about the case. On this particular occasion, the attending physician was the second-ranking surgeon in the department. I was a third-year medical student, the last person in line right behind the pathology intern and the fourth-year students.

The case was that of a woman who'd had a noncancerous lump on her thyroid gland removed from her neck. The Department Chairman asked how many different things could have gone wrong for this woman after elective surgery in such a sensitive area. The attending surgeon explained that the patient had asked to have the surgery done for cosmetic reasons. The Chairman shot back, "What are you going to do if the patient in the next room says to you, 'Doctor, I don't like my right leg anymore. Could you just take it off for me?'" The tension was palpable. There was no place to hide, not even for the most highly trained doctor.

Years later, I learned that this type of exchange was an example of the "hidden curriculum" which socializes medical students into the worst aspects of medicine. Situations like this teach students to be cynical and insensitive when it comes to the emotions of others. While surgery itself fascinated me, and I might have considered that as a specialty, there was one major problem. At our school, no surgery resident had ever entered the program married and graduated still married to the same person. My dad had also practiced surgery and was gone from home all the time. I didn't want that life for myself.

Without financial support from my family, I was determined to be self-sufficient and stay out of debt. It seemed like we were always short of money and had to find creative ways to provide for ourselves. Diane worked at a bank and then in the food service at University Hospitals where I frequently joined her for dinner. She had been working on improving my diet since we first met. Then, my lunch involved a highly nutritious Hostess fruit pie and a glass of soda. I assured Diane that this must be healthy, as the pie had some fruit in it. She disabused me of this notion by dissecting a pie right before my eyes one lunchtime. To my chagrin, there wasn't a single cherry in the entire so-called cherry fruit pie.

University Hospitals changed my eating habits for good with their special salad bar deal in which they charged by the size of the plate. A small plate cost one dollar whereas a full-size plate could be had for two dollars. A creative approach to our ever-tight budget involved ordering a small plate and then filling it with as much food as possible. We would carefully arrange the food to increase the diameter of the plate. Time for the basic principles of physics and algebra. Starting with a seven-inch plate, one places carrot and celery sticks radiating outward like spokes. The plate enlarges to nine or ten inches in size. The carrots and celery are anchored with something heavier like cottage cheese or cucumber slices. These could then be covered with peaches and other fruits and then a salad with cheese and any other offerings in the center. In those days, I would typically douse the whole thing with Thousand Island dressing. Thanks to enterprising students like us, the school eventually changed their plan where salads would be paid for by weight not by plate size.

Becoming a pediatrician

The big task of the fourth year of medical school is to secure a residency position for further training. I found that pediatric training looked much more favorable for persons seeking a balance between work and family life, so I applied to several training programs in the Midwest and West. Diane and I planned an interviewing trip to visit some great pediatric programs on a camping trip through the Dakotas and Montana before starting the circuit of residency applications on the west coast. After a visit to Stanford, we headed toward Las Vegas to see family. The whole route was designed to retrace our honeymoon in reverse order.

We were driving on an unfinished stretch of Interstate talking about the interview, excited about the prospect of studying pediatrics at a prestigious hospital. Abruptly, an oncoming driver turned right into our lane. The head on collision demolished our car, but we were unharmed. There we were in central California with all our camping gear and no way to get it all home. We found a drive-away service that needed to have a car driven to Minneapolis. We loaded our belongings into the car and canceled all the rest of my interviews except for the one in Salt Lake City, my top choice for residency outside of Madison.

Finally, the day for a decision was at hand. My two top choices were similar in many respects; both were small, highly regarded and associated with major universities. I was confident that I would be accepted at both programs so the decision was up to me. In those days, the match was conducted by filling out a card and mailed it to a central office where the students and programs would be matched. I filled out my card and put it in the mail holder at our apartment. We would be staying in Madison close to home, family and familiar surroundings. But something told us this wasn't our best option. Wouldn't it be better for us if we try something new and different? Didn't we love the West and didn't Salt Lake City also have a dietetics program where Diane could finish her training? I ran down to the mailbox, retrieved my application card, reversed the order of my preferences and then ran back to the mailbox. The mailman was there to take the envelope from my hand. There'd be no more second-guessing now. Months later, we were excited to find that I matched into the program at the University of Utah and Primary Children's Hospital. How different would our lives have been had the mailman come even a few minutes earlier?

I think of my residency days as some of the best of my entire career. It was exciting to learn new things and develop greater skills almost every day. There were so many remarkable experiences it's hard to list them all: flights for life to transport critically ill patients, the child who drowned in an icy river but was resuscitated, another child from Wyoming whose car was struck by a train, and countless sick newborns in need of newborn intensive care. Head injuries were a major problem related to any number of different kinds of accidents. I had my own accident once while attending a traveling clinic with my cardiology professor. We had just finished our final outreach clinic on a circuit through Montana and were headed back to Salt Lake City. I was driving and hit a patch of black ice, rolling the professor's car into a ditch. We both were wearing our seatbelts, and I still remember being suspended in the upside-down car. Apart from my pride, we escaped uninjured.

Pediatric residency combines hospital and clinic experiences to equip the pediatrician to care for almost any problem from birth through about age eighteen (currently up to the early twenties). The newborn intensive care unit experience was exhausting as we often worked up to thirty hour shifts every other day for six weeks at a time. This involved arriving at the hospital around 7am and leaving the following day around 1pm, assuming there were no emergencies requiring extra manpower. Other rotations were not as grueling, only requiring staying in the hospital every third or fourth night. It's hard to describe what it's like trying to sleep in a call room knowing that at any moment, a phone call could summon you to a life threatening emergency. Some people can get real rest under these circumstances, but not me. I don't think my sleep ever recovered from those nights of constant vigilance.

In the pediatric unit, residents were charged with caring for the most seriously ill children who were often transferred from outlying community hospitals. The patients usually arrived at the hospital in the afternoon or evening and were first assessed by a medical student and an intern. A more senior resident would oversee their care. The following morning, the team of trainees would present their findings to the attending physician on rounds who then conducted a teaching conference on the day's cases.

Once, we had a particularly challenging patient with chronic headaches that had developed in the hospital for no apparent reason. Neither extensive questions nor a complete battery of tests could identify the cause of his symptoms. Making my rounds at breakfast time, I noticed the patient cracking a hard-boiled egg on his forehead, precisely where his headaches were most severe. Changing his breakfast habits had a remarkable positive effect on his headaches!

Some of the patients we cared for were heart-breaking, suffering from fatal genetic conditions or incurable birth defects. I don't think I ever really appreciated how hard this must have been for the families. My focus was on understanding and treating the physiological abnormalities that would ultimately lead to the demise of these young patients. This loss of sensitivity to the human side of medicine is a common feature of American medical training, and it was happening to me.

Medical education and training involves learning a great deal of specialized knowledge, developing technical skills, and nurturing humanistic attitudes. I had grown in the areas of knowledge and skills, but, in the process, my attitudes toward patients had suffered. Like many students, the pressure and competition left little time for thoughtfulness and compassion. It became harder to see the patients and their families as real persons and not just interesting cases to be dissected, observed, and analyzed.

For me, the human side of medicine was highlighted in the continuity clinics. Run by the residents under the supervision of faculty, the clinics allow the inexperienced doctor an opportunity to take responsibility for direct patient care. Here, I learned a skill that was to become a feature of my practice for the remainder of my career. Examine children eye to eye, whether they rested on the parent's lap or the exam table. Not only did this facilitate an effective exam but it also showed respect for the child. Thanks, Dr. Marty Palmer, for teaching me to respect children at their own level.

I'd like to think that everything would work out for a doctor who is conscientious and diligent in providing patient care. Unfortunately, that's not always the case. One of the greatest challenges of my residency came the night a severely ill infant was brought to the Emergency Department. After taking the history and performing the physical exam, I reviewed the list of the most likely causes for the baby's critical condition, noting that the cardiac exam seemed normal except for weak pulses. I concluded that a severe infection was most likely the explanation and proceeded to do a spinal tap as part of the infection workup. The baby stopped breathing during the procedure and was quickly resuscitated. The tests for infection were negative, and further evaluation revealed that the initial symptoms had been caused by a narrowing of the aorta, not by an infection.

I was dismayed that following all my training, I still arrived at the wrong diagnosis and questioned whether I'd ever be qualified to care for critically ill children after this experience. My confidence was badly shaken but restored by my attending physician who reminded me that there will be times when our best efforts will still be met with unfavorable outcomes. The best I could do was to learn from these experiences and accept that no amount of effort guarantees being right all the time.

During residency, I moonlighted to help pay our bills and to make it possible for us to purchase our first house. My job was to provide continuity of care for a group of developmentally disabled persons at the American Fork Training School south of Salt Lake City. Every month, I traveled to the Training School for a Saturday morning clinic where I met my cohort of patients, reviewed their medical records, performed a brief physical exam, and made any recommendations for their general medical care. On one occasion, I had just finished a physical exam on the last patient when a new nurse joined me for the remainder of my shift. Tossing the tongue depressor into the garbage, I commented that I had been able to make it through an entire morning with just one tongue depressor. Her pale face told me she didn't realize that I was joking.

We usually had lunch in the training school cafeteria along with the school's residents, some of whom lived in cottages or group homes. One day, as I was sitting at lunch, a man sat across from me with his tray and inquired if I were a resident. I proudly answered yes, to which he stated, "I'm a resident too! Which cottage do you live in?" A lesson in humility.

I was asked to stay on at the residency program to become chief resident, a position close to junior faculty status. The program leaders felt I would be well suited for this responsibility, as I had already received the residency teaching award. By every measure, I was well-qualified but I lacked the confidence to accept the offer.

My medical school education had been largely funded by a health profession scholarship through the US Air Force and now it was time to pay them back. I could have deferred my Air Force service for the Chief Residency year, but I wanted to start seeing patients in practice. It didn't occur to me at the time that I was leaving behind the opportunity of a lifetime, nor did I consider how this decision would change the direction of my career.

Chapter 10

Developing Confidence and Humility

This is what the Lord says: "Let not the wise boast of their wisdom or the strong boast of their strength or the rich boast of their riches, but let the one who boasts boast about this: that they have the understanding to know me, that I am the Lord, who exercises kindness, justice and righteousness on earth, for in these I delight," declares the Lord.

Jeremiah 9:23-24 (NIV)

Humbled

A mother came into the Air Force Pediatric Clinic with several overly active children. Up and down they noisily jumped on and off the exam table, in spite of their mother's best efforts to control them. I was getting frustrated and having a hard time getting the history straight. Which child was she even talking about? Which one was I supposed to examine? I was getting annoyed with the disorder in my generally well-ordered routine. And they were throwing me off my schedule. Then the mother made a comment, "The problem is—"

Before she could finish her statement, I interrupted with self-justification. “The problem is that you have all these children, and I can’t take care of the one with the appointment.”

“Actually, the problem is that my husband left us today, and I don’t know where to go or what to do.”

Then my conscience and humanity entered the exam room for a lightning-fast self-talk. People sometimes say their life flashes before their eyes in a moment of grave danger: an accident, a heart attack, a near miss. I had just betrayed everything my family upbringing and years of training had taught me with my insensitivity. Clearly, this was a turning point in the making, one of those rare moments, after which one is never quite the same.

After a genuine apology for my rude treatment of this hurting mother and her children, I connected them with social services. For me, that was just the start, the straightforward part. Not so easy was the painful acceptance that my attitude was responsible for the way I handled this incident. I valued my time and sense of control over their needs. This mom and her children were being abandoned. Hadn’t I been there myself growing up in a single-parent home?

Some experiences change our perspectives; others change us more deeply. That visit was the starting point for change where it was most needed, in my heart. I resolved that I would never treat patients with such dismissiveness and sense of superiority. I needed to be a more attentive listener. I’m thankful for that experience at the beginning of my career. My patients since then have been the beneficiaries of the humbling I experienced that day. How often might doctors take a different perspective on their patients if they would only take the time to find out the patient’s real concerns and needs?

Finally practicing medicine

Finally, my first real job after over two decades of school and training came as a pediatrician serving in the U.S. Air Force. My family doesn't have much of a history of service in the armed forces. To the contrary, my ancestors were draft dodgers in Poland in the 19th century. Dad was in medical school during World War II; Mom worked in a factory supporting the war effort. I had chosen the Air Force, thinking it would give the best chance to travel and see the world. After all, they had lots of planes and service members could catch a hop for a nominal fee and travel to any base around the world. How ironic that my active duty assignment would be at the only Air Force base that didn't have planes.

Our clinic provided pediatric care for dependents of active duty and retired military personnel. During my time in the Air Force, I met some of the best doctors and nurses with whom I've ever had the privilege of working. Dr. Tom Williams was a pediatrician from Indiana who went on to teach at a medical school after his time in the Air Force. We shared clinic responsibilities, talked about cases, and brought out the best in each other's practices. In addition to the pediatricians, the clinic was staffed by the first nurse practitioners I had ever encountered. I've had a favorable impression of nurse practitioners ever since. I thoroughly enjoyed this practice setting where I could care for patients without all the responsibility of running the clinic.

Providing medical center-level care for children in a small hospital was a real challenge for a newly trained physician. I thought the medical skills I had so painstakingly acquired in training would be the key to my success. Of course, those skills were necessary, but they weren't enough. To practice quality medicine, I needed a complete team including trained nurses, anesthesiology, surgery, lab, X-Ray, to name just a few. All these others worked behind the scenes; the doctor got most of the attention.

In the Air Force, the pilots got the attention, praise and recognition. They're the ones with the stories to tell of their dramatic work. Not so for the mechanics, technicians, and countless others (It's said that each pilot is supported by up to 100 persons) who make the pilot's flight possible. I saw my position as the most important one on the medical team and took other team members for granted. Slowly, I realized that it takes more than a well-trained doctor to provide excellent medical care. Unfortunately, I forgot this important lesson as my career advanced.

Life in the pediatric clinic

In the pediatric clinic, I had the opportunity to meet many appreciative families. Sometimes, though, the families made what I considered to be unreasonable requests. On one occasion, I was at the front desk when a mother rushed into the clinic holding a small bottle of ear drops. "Could I use these ear drops on my daughter? She's having some ear problems."

"Tell me more about the drops."

The woman responded irately that the drops were prescribed for the family cat and questioned how much trouble they could cause her daughter. I tried to inform her that we don't normally recommend giving medicine prescribed for pets to our children. She didn't want to talk about that and stormed out the door.

It was a joy for me to meet so many families and provide care for their children. Sometimes, the pediatric encounters were humorous like the time I was speaking with the father of a four-month-old baby. I had commented that the baby seemed to be happy and good natured, to which the father responded, "Happy! When we're watching TV together, he'll be jawing on a French fry, and laugh at the jokes before I do." I wasn't sure what to make of the infant's quick appreciation of humor, but I did try to point out that French fries are probably not the ideal food for an infant.

At the Air Force hospital, members of the medical staff took turns covering the Emergency Room at night and on weekends. An older woman was brought to the ER by her daughter after passing out on the couch while clipping coupons. The thought crossed my mind that this must have been quite a valuable coupon but, this was a life-threatening situation and it demanded immediate action. I initiated evaluation measures including placing a cardiac monitor and then contacted the internist on call for further guidance. While I was on the phone, the patient's daughter rushed into the nurses' station. Motioning with her hand, she asked me, "What does it mean when that line on the screen that goes up and down all of a sudden goes flat?"

I dashed into the room to find the patient's anxious eyes wide open. The cardiac monitor showed a flat tracing indicating that her heart had stopped even though she was still conscious and alert. I grabbed her shoulders and shook her to see if she could respond when her heartbeat suddenly resumed without any further medication or treatment. I can guarantee that if I myself had been attached to a cardiac monitor, the line on my screen would have been rapidly going up and down. The internist rushed in from home and arranged for the woman to have an emergency pacemaker placed that night.

My most challenging ER experience was the case of a young woman who came in with a butcher knife stuck into her abdomen. Her boyfriend stated that an accident had occurred when she'd tripped and fallen while carrying a knife down the steps. The woman was in shock and only barely conscious, the entire blade of a large knife buried in her abdomen and only the handle visible. I inserted the largest IV lines I had ever seen so we could pour blood and other fluids into her circulation as fast as possible. The surgeon was called in. His first instruction was to leave the knife alone. During the surgery, the bleeding was halted, and the knife was found to be stuck into the inner aspect of her pelvis with its tip bent. This was no accidental fall; she had been stabbed! Despite all of our resuscitation efforts, the woman died in surgery from massive blood loss. The boyfriend was arrested and brought to justice.

Becoming a 'second victim"

The most traumatic experience of my Air Force career centered around two siblings who died from head injuries about two years apart. When the first child was found to have a skull fracture, the family was thoroughly investigated, and no indication of child abuse was discovered. That child subsequently died from problems associated with a brain injury. When the family's second child died under similar circumstances, another child abuse investigation followed.

Since the second event had occurred on an Air Force Base, the FBI conducted the investigation. The neighbors reported that they had heard shouting and yelling in the family's home on many occasions. I was summoned to testify at the mother's trial in Federal Court where she was found guilty of murdering her two infant children. She had an underlying emotional health condition and was sentenced to a long prison sentence. An outcome like this would cause any doctor to re-examine the case step by step. I began to experience self-doubt about my ability to look out for my patients. Had I overlooked some subtle warning? Hadn't I followed all the right steps in looking out for the welfare of these children? Was there some key clue I had missed?

I felt like I had done my best for the children. I had sought medical consultation about the injuries. I had followed all the rules in reporting suspected child abuse and cooperating with any investigations that were taking place. Tragically, even doing one's best isn't always enough to ensure the right outcome. In a sense, I saw this whole experience as a failure on my part and one which shook my confidence in my ability to accurately assess the needs of my patients.

In recent years, there's been increasing interest in the way caring for victims of trauma or violence impacts the caregivers who essentially become "second victims." Being involved in health care exacts a toll on members of the medical team. Unfortunately, this only came to be understood around the end of my medical career.

A similar blow to my confidence occured in my residency when a critically ill infant patient of mine almost died. Fortunately, an attending physician helped me through this by reminding me that a physician will sometimes have a bad outcome in spite of their best efforts. Once I was on my own in practice, there was no mentor in whom I could confide. Doctors don't talk about their near misses or bad outcomes. They mostly hope nobody will find out.

Practicing medicine involves more than seeing patients; administrative responsibilities await the physician at every turn. The commanders at our hospital soon recognized that I had a knack for administration. No one told me to be wary about excelling at these kinds of tasks. Before long, I started getting assigned to take over other doctors' committee work. One doctor routinely took the day off when he was to chair a committee we served on. As the second ranking officer, the leadership responsibility fell to me.

Life in the military isn't for everyone, especially professionals who take pride in thinking for themselves and making independent decisions. Many times, we were instructed to follow orders based on drills and training scenarios. One time, the entire clinic staff spent the better part of a clinic day sitting in an inside hallway to simulate our response in the event of a nuclear attack at a nearby base. The Air Force was paying my salary, so if they wanted me to sit in the hallway for a day, it was their right.

That was an important day for me, as it forced me to consider my loyalty to my role as an Air Force physician. Someone with more information and a broader perspective than I had made the decision about this drill and ensured no patients would suffer from the staff's participation in the drill. For me, the exercise was about being a team player, willing to follow orders without complaining.

By the end of my four years of active duty, I received the Meritorious Service Award, had been promoted to Major and was on my way to a successful military career. Extending my Air Force service would involve relocating our family, now numbering three children under the age of five to another base. Things might have been different if I had gotten the assignment I was looking for at Ellsworth Air Force Base in Anchorage Alaska, but that option wasn't available. Continuing on in the Air Force would also have necessitated taking on more administrative responsibilities, and I wanted to see patients full time. Staying in the Air Force would also have required several moves. Diane and I decided to decline the Air Force's offer. As it turned out, we moved more on our own than the Air Force would ever have required, often at our own expense. I am thankful that I was able to serve our country in the military and stand proudly when active duty and retired service members are acknowledged at church or other settings.

Four years out of residency, I was ready to find a stable, connected life for my family. I had received excellent training and had paid back my Air Force commitment. I was ready to return home where my dream job awaited me, only it turned out to be a different type of dream than I anticipated.

Chapter 11

From dream to nightmare

For you created my inmost being; You knit me together in my mother's womb. I praise you because I am fearfully and wonderfully made.

Psalm 139:13-14 (NIV)

Returning with my wife and three children to practice in my hometown was the fulfillment of a long-standing dream to practice medicine in the clinic my father had started. This was the community where I'd grown up and would be caring for "my people." After years away, we would now be surrounded by our extended families. This was home, where I first sat in the car while my dad made house calls, where I paraded around the hospital in Dad's pants and played hide and seek in the basement. I had done research in one hospital during college and lived for a month in another during a medical school rotation. Now I could put my years of training and practice experience to use in the clinic, hospital, newborn nursery, and Emergency Department. A long and successful career awaited me.

How old do you have to be to get married?

I loved practicing Pediatrics with its challenge of relating to children at one level and to their parents at another. It might seem more efficient to restrict the talk in patient visits to the parents who have most of the information we're looking for. But parents can't tell us all we need to know. Even young children can provide a lot of valuable information about their home, family life, and personal health concerns if given the opportunity. They just need to be treated respectfully and with a certain measure of playfulness.

To open a patient visit, I asked a five-year-old boy one of my favorite questions, "Are you married yet?"

"No! I'm too young to get married. I'm only five."

"How old do you need to be to get married?"

"Six. I've got the girl picked out."

"Where are you going to live? How are you going to support yourselves?"

"We're going to live in a trailer in the driveway. She'll go to work, and I'll stay home watching TV."

I always had a special place in my heart for families under duress, sometimes from limited financial means, other times from lack of skills or abilities. Single parent families were also a special concern. Many times, these families were judged harshly for having Medical Assistance insurance. Other times, they might be self-conscious of their old clothing or general appearance. One day a couple came to receive care for their niece, a toddler. They had no insurance and their clothes looked old and worn out. After the visit, they asked how they were to settle their bill. In a burst of good will, I assured them that there would be no charge. After all, they were doing so much themselves by taking in the young child. I felt proud of my generosity until a nurse asked me if I knew the couple. The man had recently signed a lucrative contract with the Packers and would make more money in the next couple of years than I would in my entire career. Though I lost out on the income from that visit, I felt more embarrassed than upset, but would rather see myself governed by a sense of compassion than one of financial gain, even if my good intentions were occasionally misdirected. Another time, I spoke out when a patient on welfare was being derided in a clinic staff discussion. It became clear that some in the clinic didn't share my altruistic perspective.

Pediatric practice is mostly devoted to daily visits for well-child care, acute care, and follow ups. Each of these were fairly predictable but rewarding in their own ways. The most dramatic activities in practice occur after-hours when the rewards and stresses were magnified. It might be easiest to understand pediatric call by putting it in contrast to current practice. In those days, being on call meant taking phone calls all night. Call meant covering the emergency room and being available for deliveries. Weekends required hospital rounds on the pediatric floor and in the newborn nursery. All this took place after the pediatrician would have been working in the clinic all day or all week. It was a recipe for mistakes and bad outcomes.

Today, a triage nurse takes care of the phone calls. In the hospital, children are cared for by Emergency Department specialists and Pediatric Hospitalists; Neonatologists attend high-risk deliveries and cover the Neonatal Intensive Care Unit. These are all backed up with ready access to transport services, always on standby in the event of life-threatening emergencies. None of these services were available at my main hospital during my time in pediatric practice.

Emergency situations provided some of my strongest recollections from my days in pediatric practice. I was on call in the emergency room the evening some children were playing in a quarry and tried to dig a cave into the bottom of a sandpile. The sand collapsed and one of the children suffocated. Resuscitation efforts failed. All I could do was sit with the grieving family after informing them of their child's death until they could be ministered to by the chaplain and surrounded by supportive family and friends. But in those days, no one talked with the doctors, nurses, and other members of the medical team after a tragedy like this. No one prepared them for when they went home to their own children who might be the same age as the child who had just died. No one cared for the caregivers.

Many primary care physicians find some medical conditions to be particularly interesting. For me, it was the care of children with asthma. In my pediatric residency, a dynamic allergist showed me that taking care of children with asthma could be very rewarding. When I later entered practice in the Air Force, we saw many children with asthma and allergies. That's to be expected, as approximately 20% of children have symptoms related to these conditions. We invited an allergist from a nearby base to conduct a consultation clinic at our hospital. He helped us provide the best care for our patients and taught us about asthma and allergy care. I didn't realize it at the time, but this approach was to become the foundation for my future outreach efforts into our community. The best use of a consultant was to provide excellent care and then train the caregivers to do the same in their own practices.

More and more, I wanted to care for patients with asthma and allergy related conditions. But without the training or credentials, how could I do this? My first solution was to take a three-week mini-fellowship at the University of Wisconsin. There, I learned to take a detailed history. Knowledge of lung function and skin testing completed this short training. I was now ready to provide a broader range of services for my patients. Or so I thought. It's one thing to provide this care for children, but allergy often runs in families. Children with allergies tend to have allergic parents and several of them asked me to be their doctor too, almost like a family allergy practice. This challenged my clinic's mindset and caused considerable tension with my partners who insisted that we were strictly a Pediatric clinic. The parents would have to find somewhere else to receive their care.

I had seen how my dad devoted himself to his patients, and I wanted to follow his example of dedicated service to others. At the same time, I had also experienced the downside of growing up in a medical household with an overly busy doctor who was often absent from home. I wanted to avoid becoming that kind of doctor for the sake of my own family. These goals didn't have to be irreconcilable, but in my Green Bay practice setting, they were.

As tensions grew, I gradually found myself responding to work-related situations out of fear rather than collegiality. This hit home when I remained at work the day of my favorite uncle's funeral, afraid to ask for time off. Things got even worse when I inquired about the possibility of taking paternity leave with our next pregnancy. In those days, male physicians never did that. My request was interpreted as a sign of weakness and lack of dedication to my patients, my practice, and my partners. My dream of hometown practice was unraveling around me, even though I had done everything I could to build a successful practice. It wasn't good enough. Something would need to change.

A nightmare tests my faith

You intended to harm me, but God intended it for good.

Genesis 50: 20 (NIV)

Up to this time, things had been going according to the career schedule I had developed years earlier: do well in school, get the right residency training, satisfy your obligations to the Air Force, and return home to practice. Those were my objectives and I had achieved them, but they had been accomplished before I had a sense of God's role in my life. How would I know if I had achieved this on my own abilities, or was God somehow involved?

At home, faith was at the center of how we were going to raise our children, with a combination of Bible teachings, devotions and spiritual practices like mealtime prayers, Advent devotions, and church attendance. We tried to follow the advice offered by Christian radio speakers and assumed that doing the right activities would result in good outcomes. At this point, the life of faith didn't seem very demanding, but I began to question whether my spiritual beliefs could withstand serious challenges. After all, things were looking pretty good for me with my secure medical practice, thriving family, and improving financial condition. I naively prayed, "Lord, test me so I can know if my faith is real." Be careful what you pray for.

It didn't take long for my prayer to be answered.

We were getting ready to visit our friends in Ohio for the long Fourth of July holiday weekend. Just one-half day of clinic to go before our vacation. A staff member delivered a message about a management meeting to take place after clinic hours. I thought the meeting would be about the proposed changes in our medical records system.

I walked into a tense meeting room where the clinic president, clinic manager, a board member, and the senior member of my department were awaiting my arrival. Something didn't feel right. Why was this group meeting to talk about the medical record system? Several of them weren't even on the committee. I took my seat in silence, mouth dry, stomach churning, heart pounding. One by one each person delivered their summary judgment:

"You're a danger to your patients and a liability to the clinic."

""It doesn't matter if you are a member of the clinic. You'll never practice here again."

"There's nothing you can do to change this decision."

"No patient is going to follow you if you stay in town."

"Maybe you should think about leaving Green Bay."

"Maybe you should think about quitting medicine altogether."

My mind raced as my professional identity was shredded. No one had ever expressed concern about my performance before this, and here I was being fired on the spot. What had happened to turn my dream into a nightmare?

A few weeks earlier, a critically ill baby had come into the Emergency Room with features of a bowel obstruction. Making this diagnosis was the easy part. Getting the needed care was impossible. I had tried to transfer the baby to the newborn intensive care unit across town for further care, but they were full. We had nowhere else to send the baby and transfer out of the community wasn't possible at that time.

The surgeon on call at our community hospital was certain he had the technical skill to perform the delicate surgery. Unfortunately, we didn't have the right resources, like pediatric anesthesia and skilled neonatal intensive care nursing to support the baby during and after surgery. I tried to suggest that the baby's surgery be done elsewhere but was outranked on the clinical team. I was in the operating room to be ready for the patient's recovery. The surgery was a success, but the baby's condition quickly worsened. I needed backup and called one of my partners for help. In spite of all our efforts, the baby succumbed to shock in the postoperative period. I was crushed by this entire experience, the loss of this patient, the impossible situation I had been put into, my failure to stand up for the patient's best interests.

This was a devastating blow to my self-image as a competent and caring physician. I had devoted over a decade of my life after college to becoming a physician and now was being declared incompetent by my peers. As a full member of the clinic, this dismissal violated all my rights as part owner of the clinic. Regardless of that, I would never practice in that group again. When the case was later reviewed by a group of pediatricians, no fault was found in my care, but that didn't change the decision at the clinic. I was out.

My confidence was badly shaken, and I was now out of a job with three children and a fourth on the way. My dream of practicing in my dad's clinic was shattered. What would I do next? With no advance preparation, I would need to establish an independent solo pediatric practice. Leaving town or abandoning medicine were not options. But first, I had to restore my confidence.

I sought the help of a staff psychiatrist who likened my experience to a mugging in which each member of the gang got in a punch or a hard kick and then left me in the gutter to die. I was careful to ensure that these visits were not public knowledge. Hospital credentials committees and governing boards still take a dim view of the doctor who seeks help for emotional concerns.

While between jobs, I got to thinking about how we often long for time off when we're busy at work. However, having lots of free time doesn't seem like much of a vacation for the unemployed. Not even severance pay compensates for the embarrassment and shame of getting fired, the uncertainties of supporting a family, the questions of competence and self-worth. Through this experience, I gained a new appreciation for the struggles of those out of work, especially when their unemployment occurs under unfair circumstances.

Within a month, with the help of family and friends, my solo pediatric practice was up and running. I found space in the same building as my old office, only one floor down. Eventually, more than 600 of my former patients followed me to my new office. When they called my former clinic to transfer their care, they were frequently told no one knew how I could be found. Even coming to the same building didn't help them locate me as my name was repeatedly scratched off the nameplate on the elevator.

Practicing in the same building, I ran into my former partners on a regular basis. To say that this was uncomfortable would be an understatement. When I realized that none of the other pediatricians in town wanted to get involved with the internal affairs of my prior clinic, I knew I'd need to rethink my career plans to practice in my hometown. I could handle solo practice and be on call almost every night, but I would never leave medicine.

With my new clinic established, I was free to practice without having critical associates looking over my shoulder all the time. I was free to express my sense of humor and enjoy being a doctor once again. I also had the opportunity to begin consulting for the Oneida Tribe at their Health Care Center, in a sense, fulfilling my dad's dream of serving the Native American population.

It's one thing to appreciate the big picture spiritual impact of a painful event like this and to see the unanticipated benefits. I knew that traumatic experiences leave a lasting impact, and I believed that something meant for evil can turn out for our good. Neither of these truths takes away the pain, the guilt, and the self doubt of the event itself.

Life events like getting fired have consequences and I resolved that I would never trust anyone again with my work-related welfare. I had hit the bottom and resolved to never give anyone the power or opportunity to abandon me. I had been let down in childhood and now again as an adult. I began to question whether I could trust anyone in the workplace. Unfortunately, this mindset would have negative effects on my work life for years to come. Although I had been able to open a new medical practice, I would need more than my own strength if I were ever going to have a successful long-term career. While my extended family, friends, and professional colleagues helped me make it back to work on my own, I never doubted that it was my faith and Diane's unwavering support that got me through this time.

One of the joys of studying the Bible is the way we learn about how Biblical figures responded when they came under pressure. In my journal entries made at the time I was fired, I recorded how I took consolation from the Old Testament story of Joseph and his brothers (now popularized in the play, *Joseph and his Amazing Technicolor Dreamcoat)*. In this story, Joseph's jealous brothers sold him into slavery. Unbeknownst to them, Joseph rose to become second-in-command of the entire nation of Egypt. When a severe famine occurred, the brothers sought food in Egypt, Joseph oversaw the food distribution. The one they had sold as a slave now had the power of life and death over them. The brothers feared for their lives until Joseph reassured them. "You meant this for evil, but God meant it for good."

Years later, I ran into one of the physicians from my personal firing squad and we finally had a conversation. I had seen him at hospital meetings, but always had avoided talking with him. The pain and sense of betrayal from that meeting dominated my thinking. I saw the clinic's action as an attempt to ruin me and my family. The doctor's recollection of the event was completely different. He acknowledged that concerns about patient care were only the pretext for the real issue. My desire for a balanced life was at odds with the prevailing culture of the clinic. Firing me was basically a way to placate the members of my department. They were more valuable to the clinic than I was.

Getting fired was the faith-testing event that I had prayed for, so in a sense, it was an answer to prayer. I learned first hand that my faith was real. God would never abandon me.

We had survived the major assault on my career and our family when I was railroaded out of that job. What I didn't realize at the time was that trials like this prepare us for even greater tests in the future. For me, these were going to involve the hopes and dreams I cherished most dearly: the desire to have a stable and happy family and a marriage that could last a lifetime.

Chapter 12

A Fresh Start

Remember not the former things, nor consider the things of old. Behold I am doing a new thing, now it springs forth, do you not perceive it? I will make a way in the wilderness and rivers in the desert.

Isaiah 43:18-19 (ESV)

Another move/more training/a new job

When I was growing up, workers often remained on the same job for life. That's not how my dad approached his work nor the way I would pursue my career either. I developed the notion that some type of career move every seven to ten years would keep my thinking fresh. The Renaissance Man from high school was now the restless doctor on the job. By the time we had our fifth child, we had moved five times for my work or school.

The positive side of all this moving around was that I was able to work with some great people, receive great training and live in some great places. But I never gave much thought to the cost to our family and the impact it would have on me over time. I had grown up in a stable neighborhood, but my children weren't able to have the same experience. The frequent moves, school changes, and the need to repeatedly make and then leave friends took a great toll on them and even more so on Diane.

For fifteen years, I had devoted myself to my medical education, training and pediatric practice and thought I had arrived at my destination of a stable home, family, and work setting. Only I had been wrong. Rebounding from getting fired, I started a new practice but the 24/7 call would be impossible to sustain for long. I began praying for a new direction for my career, and applied to allergy fellowship programs around the country. This process usually took two or three years. I could have simply called myself an allergist without the training, but was determined to hold myself to the highest standard of fellowship training.

It didn't take long for my prayers to be answered through a life-changing phone call. Dr. William Busse, head of the Allergy Training Program at the University of Wisconsin, asked if I would consider coming to Madison for an allergy fellowship in a couple of months to fill an unexpected opening. Diane and I talked it over at lunch and decided to accept the offer. We then tried to imagine how we could be ready to move to Madison on such short notice..

Over the next several weeks, we had to make arrangements that could easily take a year. The pediatric practice had to be closed, patients transferred to other clinics and medical records stored. We closed out the financial books, found housing in Madison, and sold our house in Green Bay. Next came arranging to move, finishing out the school year, and enrolling the kids in a school in Madison. With four children and the youngest only six months old, this was a tremendous strain on Diane who worked more than full time as a stay at home mom.

I had always loved being in school and looked forward to the new adventure.but I didn't anticipate the challenge of going from the autonomy of solo practice to the regimented life of fellowship training. On my first day of fellowship, I arrived about five minutes late to the Allergy Clinic where I would work with Dr. Busse himself. There he stood at the door, silently looking at his watch. No words needed. I was never late again for one of his clinics.

The fellowship was an amazing time of learning the subject of allergy and asthma care from world authorities. I didn't appreciate at the time just how prominent the UW Allergy Department was with its world-renowned faculty, specialists who wrote the allergy textbooks and were leaders of international medical societies. Studying under them was a unique privilege that came from an unexpected phone call.

The fellowship provided opportunities to do clinical research. The most interesting topic we studied was that of latex allergy, a growing problem with the advent of universal precautions to prevent infectious diseases like HIV-AIDS. We were able to identify several key factors involved in this growing epidemic leading to improved efforts at prevention. The latex allergy studies received an award at a national meeting. Ordinarily, receiving such recognition for my efforts would be a great cause for celebration. The meeting was in Orlando, so we took our kids with a planned side trip to Disneyland. Our hotel vacation hopes were dashed when we learned our room was actually next door to Dr. Busse's. I spent most of my time trying to keep the kids quiet and avoid his constant surveillance. After the award ceremony, we moved to a different hotel.

One of the remarkable things about training at a renowned Medical Center is the diversity and complexity of patients seen by the world-class specialists. I became impressed by the number of people from Green Bay who traveled all the way to Madison for specialized allergy care. Many of them could have been cared for locally if only adequately trained doctors could be found. Perhaps I could be the one to provide that care were I to return home.

Several specific patients had quite an impact on me. One man was suffering from chronic sinus infections felt to be related to allergy or immune deficiency. Extensive testing failed to identify the cause of his problems, so he came to our clinic for further evaluation. "What do you like to do for hobbies?" I asked. "Water skiing," he replied. The jet spray of water from the water skiing constantly assaulted his sinuses, leading to the repeated infections. Question answered.

An older woman came in with a history of suspected insect sting allergy. She had collapsed after a bee sting. Taking care of such a potentially life-threatening problem requires a detailed history. The original story was that the woman was stung by a bee and then felt faint and almost collapsed. Going over her history minute by minute, the story changed. She had been mowing her backyard and felt a little faint from the heat and exertion. On her way into the house to rest, she was stung by a bee. Concerned, she called her daughter for help. While the daughter was en route, the woman proceeded out into the front yard to finish cutting the grass before the paramedics arrived. Thankfully, her allergy tests were negative; she had just over-exerted herself. No harm done, save a little embarrassment.

Sometimes, a poem will pop into my head when I'm struck by an unusual circumstance. If I sense an emotional connection with the patient, I might share this with them as in this case:

Here I lie, dead and gone;

but at least I finished my front lawn.

I found the mix of work in the clinic, lab, and library an almost perfect combination for someone like myself. I liked the professional stimulation that came from leaders in my field, conferences of interest and research. I even had opportunities to teach medical students and residents. At the conclusion of my fellowship, I was asked to consider staying on with the Department as a clinical instructor but, instead, moved back to Salt Lake City to join a private allergy practice with teaching opportunities where I had studied Pediatrics.

This is the place

I had received several job offers to return to Green Bay but none were right for me. I wanted to be my own person and practice in a way that reflected my belief in personalized patient care. We moved back to Salt Lake City in 1990 where I joined Intermountain Allergy Clinic, at the time, one of the largest allergy and asthma clinics in the country. I was going to practice alongside the asthma specialist I had admired during my pediatric training. Our previous experience in Salt Lake City had been great; a return seemed ideal. Unfortunately, my dreams were never quite realized upon our return to Utah.

Shortly after our arrival in Salt Lake City, I was assigned to attend an asthma camp at Snowbird Resort where children with asthma would be taught self-management skills. Games and physical activities reinforced the teaching lessons. Health-related camps are popular for children with chronic conditions. I had prior experience with diabetes camps during my pediatric residency and the asthma camp was something I looked forward to: a new way to teach important concepts and skills to empower patients.

The Snowbird Asthma Camp was going well until a camper tripped while running down the ski hill and suffered a cut on his head. I was the camp doctor staying at the resort for emergencies such as this and to teach the young campers about asthma self-care. An EMT assigned to the camp was certain that we could take care of the laceration with the suture materials on hand. The injured student appeared to be fine neurologically and scalp lacerations generally tend to heal quite nicely. Something didn't seem right to me. I insisted that we take the camper to the nearest hospital. This decision was criticized by others in charge of the camp, but I held my ground. I wasn't going to let someone else's judgment override my commitment to providing the best care for a child like I had before. Never again!

I personally escorted the injured camper to the emergency room and sat in the waiting area while he was being evaluated. Following a brief assessment, the Emergency Room doctor was about to start placing the sutures when he discovered a piece of bone poking into the wound. He abruptly stopped putting in the sutures and hurried out to the waiting area with a worried look on his face. The patient had suffered an open skull fracture and needed to be hospitalized for observation and possible surgery. Thankfully, the young camper recovered completely. But he never would have if I had placed those sutures in a hotel room.

Every physician knows that a single mistake could lead to a malpractice suit. My entire medical career could have ended with one wrong decision at the ski resort. Following my instincts had saved the day. Most of the time in medicine, we make decisions based on analysis of all the factual data that's available. Other times like this, it's all about following intuition even in the face of strong opposition.

My only lawsuit

It's estimated that over half of all doctors in the United States will be cited in a malpractice suit at some point in their career. The only time this ever happened to me was related to a patient I saw in the allergy clinic in Salt Lake City. I was accused of failing to diagnose the cause of a patient's problem. It's hard to describe the shock and sense of dread that comes with a notice of a pending lawsuit and the anxious years of consultation with lawyers, depositions, and phone calls. The medical records are scrutinized for errors, misjudgments, or signs of personal failure. While the suit was eventually dropped, it continued to impact me throughout the remainder of my career. From this point on, the fact of having been cited in a lawsuit had to be disclosed on every application for hospital privileges.

Though I may have generally shown great medical judgment, the same couldn't be said for some of my family life decisions. Diane and I were still operating with the mindset that we needed to avoid debt at all costs, even if that meant making personal sacrifices. This led to the huge mistake of having only one car for our family in suburban Salt Lake City where there's no public transportation. This meant that whenever I drove to work, Diane would be relegated to staying home with Emily until I returned. My misguided efforts to save money were shortsighted. Sometimes, frugality is expensive and in this case, cost us many opportunities for Diane to become more involved in our new community.

It didn't take long for problems to surface on this new job. I was seeing more patients than I ever imagined possible and started to feel like I was part of a production line. The doctor I had emulated was rarely available, as he pursued research and his personal interests. The opportunity to teach was one of the reasons why I'd chosen the job, but teaching was reserved for the more senior doctors. Friction with our office manager developed over a number of issues related to the production mindset, and I eventually resigned out of frustration.

Once again, we needed to sell our house on fairly short notice to accomplish our move back to Green Bay.

Did it have to turn out this way? Couldn't we have worked something out so we could stay in Utah? Certainly, but I had been so bruised by my earlier clinic experiences that I didn't feel like I could trust anyone. Troubles in the clinic only confirmed that belief, but how much of this had I brought on myself? I realized much later that I saw things as I wanted to see them, and only accepted what confirmed my preconceived notions and opinions.

Our time in Salt Lake City was the final time our family life was in harmony. Our children were doing well in a great school with Rachel in sixth grade, Tony in fourth and Sam in second, Emily a preschooler at home. We had deepening friendships and worshiped in a supportive church environment with solid Bible teaching. I took all of this for granted as I made plans for the next exciting phase of my career never thinking what another move would do to our family.

And this move would be particularly difficult. Our home sold the first weekend it was listed–full price cash offer, no negotiations, closing in one week. We barely had time to pack our belongings and arrange for them to be moved. Moving back to Green Bay on short notice also meant we had to quickly find somewhere to live. Diane found a place for us to stay at the convent connected to the Chrisitian school where she would be teaching part-time. We squeezed our family into rooms formerly occupied by nuns while we looked for a more suitable home (one in which the bathroom didn't have five stalls and four tubs and showers.) By the time we found a house to move into, Diane was pregnant with Peter.

On our return trip to Green Bay, we encountered some rough weather while driving through central Wisconsin. We were listening to a sermon recorded by the new pastor of the church we were going to visit once we settled in. His style reminded us of the type of teaching we had received in the Bible Study Fellowship program. Stopping at a rest area, we were impressed with the ferocity of the winds and rain. Unbeknownst to us, a tornado had touched down in the vicinity at around the same time as our stop. The pastor's sermon was too good to interrupt for us to check on the weather. We were headed home, this time to build our lives on our own terms. Little did we realize that we were heading into a storm far greater than a tornado.

Finally home for good

We were back in Green Bay, after our second circuit through Madison and Salt Lake City and were ready to return to practice. I joked that I had everything a doctor could need for success to open an independent practice: no patients, no place to work, no staff, and no money. Only a great reputation, incredible training, a love for medicine, and a desire to serve. And a respected family name. We had so little, yet we had so much.

My practice was going to provide personalized asthma and allergy care, each aspect reflecting my spiritual beliefs. In practical terms, this meant establishing an ethical medical practice in a world where business integrity is often overlooked. This required paying bills on time and establishing retirement programs for my staff and accepting the guidance of my team of advisors. Anyone who worked in my practice would maintain a respectful tone in the office for each patient and member of our team, just as I had been taught to speak of others.

PART FOUR

FAITH TESTED

Chapter 13

Trials of family life

Consider it pure joy, my brothers and sisters, whenever you face trials of many kinds, because you know that the testing of your faith produces perseverance. Let perseverance finish its work so that you may be mature and complete, not lacking anything.

James 1: 2-4 (ESV)

How I almost ruined my marriage

For most doctors, a growing family, independent solo practice, and community involvement would be more than enough to qualify as a full life. But not for me. I felt I needed more, and I began to look for ways to stretch myself personally and professionally. This involved taking on speaking engagements for work and agreeing to join a Christian Medical and Dental Association (CMDA) trip to Hungary where I would be speaking and teaching at a children's hospital. This would prove my competence and give me something to report to others. My head swelled with images of greatness.

Diane expressed deep concern about the mission trip since Peter was less than 6 months old, but I didn't listen. Instead, I saw this decision as a matter of competing values and principles. Our pastor assured me that keeping one's word was Scriptural and people on the mission field were counting on me. But so was my family.

It's amazing how a person can rationalize almost anything when motivated by their selfish will and a poorly applied verse from the Bible. In the end, I was more concerned about what others thought and less about what my own family needed. Completely opposite of what the Bible clearly tells us. I saw the decision to travel as a reflection of my integrity and it was, only reflecting my lack of integrity. At our wedding I promised to honor my wife. Instead, I chose to pursue my own will. This has been the most regrettable decision of my life, leaving Diane, our four children and the baby behind. Where had I seen that before?

In one sense, the trip was a great success. My lectures and teaching were well-received, and I felt like I was adding a new dimension to my career: Dr. Jim Warpinski, international speaker and missionary! Several days into the trip, a phone call home brought me back to reality. With five children to watch over, Diane was overwhelmed, tearful, and angry. How could I have abandoned her like that? What kind of man leaves his wife and family behind to pursue his dreams? I canceled the remaining days of my trip and flew home. Almost prophetically, the in-flight movie, *Mrs. Doubtfire*, was a story about children of divorce, too close to home for me. Through tear-filled eyes, I could finally see clearly; I was becoming just like my dad, restless and determined to pursue my own interests. Worse, I was in the process of abandoning people I loved.

This event destroyed my hoped for image of being the ideal husband. My pride and selfish ambition had almost destroyed my marriage and family. For much of my life, I had been fearful that others would abandon me. For the first time, I realized that the greatest threat to my own marriage didn't come from the outside, it had come from within myself. If I could disregard my wife's pleading like this, what else might I be capable of? I resolved to be a more responsive listener and never travel again without Diane's approval. It was 10 years before I went on another mission trip. It took even longer before I was able to restore her trust.

Dad's bed revisited

Not long after this disastrous trip, MaryAnn called to tell me that Dad's health had taken a turn for the worse. His prostate cancer had spread and therapy was no longer working. The end was near. One by one, my siblings and I flew to Las Vegas for a final visit. Ever one to look at the bright side, Dad described it as a "Living Wake." We each shared stories with him and received his parting words of encouragement, a final blessing. Now in my mid-forties and with five children of my own, I could see firsthand the challenges of being a father. Why hadn't I ever asked him about that? What had I been afraid to learn?

That final visit with Dad forced me to face the painful event that had set my whole quest in motion. Only as he neared the end of his life could we talk about this, and I could begin to see our family life from his perspective. Dad said he felt his very life was at stake with all the pressure and discord at home and the arguing about drinking; he felt sorry that he felt he had to leave us to survive. For the first time, I was able to see beyond my own response to my parents' divorce. How different life might have been had I been bold enough to talk with him about this sooner.

Storms on the horizon

About a year after Dad's passing, I was looking out the living room window for signs of Rachel. Now sixteen years old, she had stormed out of the house in a flash of anger several hours before. She had done this once before when she threatened to run away. On that occasion, she only got as far as the front yard where she sat perched in the maple tree smoking a cigarette with a friend. This time was different. The tree was empty.

Smoking was forbidden in our home and was about the worst thing I could imagine at the time. We never did find out for sure what Rachel did for the day she was missing from home.

I never imagined there could be troubles like this in my family. I never imagined there could be issues like this in my family. The worst we boys did was sneak my uncle's cigars and burn a hole in the backseat of his car, a crime for which my mother had us each smoke an entire cigar on the back porch.

Cries for help

Nothing prepared us for what came after Rachel's brief disappearance. When her school notified us of disciplinary issues, we had to try a different approach to our parenting. Up to this time, we tolerated small acts of resistance and rebellion at home hoping they would somehow end, but they only worsened. Now Sam was starting to act out as well. I was coaching his fifth grade basketball team and instructed the players to work on their layups, free throws and passing drills. Sam ignored the rest of the team to take three-point shots. A good coach would have benched him. Unfortunately, I couldn't just bench my own kids in practices or at home.

Trusted friends and concerned school staff suggested we consider counseling as a family. Initially, I resisted, thinking I should have been able to solve the problem. Going to a counselor meant admitting that I had come up short as a parent. It meant I needed help from others, and I wasn't the kind of person who admitted someone in his family needed help. I had grown up in a culture of silence, an unspoken gag order on talking about our family problems outside the home.

I would like to say that the counseling helped us sort out all of our problems but in reality, our troubles were beyond the scope of the counselors we were seeing. Sometimes we would attend counseling as a family and leave feeling we were either too lenient or too stringent. It all depended on which counselor we happened to see that day. One counselor was certain that the problems in our family stemmed from my role as a physician. After all, he suggested, weren't doctors too busy with their work to pay attention to their own children? He didn't know how hard I had tried to be involved with our kids, volunteering to coach or help out in the classroom.

As the counseling progressed, we lost faith in the process. One counselor determined that the root of our family's problems was the strictness of our home environment. To her, our problem came from putting our Christian beliefs on parenting into action. All we had to do was relax the rules, allow more personal freedom, and wait to see the beneficial results that would follow. This went against our common sense and personal beliefs but how can untrained parents challenge a professional counselor? When this advice turned out to be an abject failure, the counselor brushed it off. "Well, let's just try the other approach of more rules and see how that works." If raising children were akin to a lab experiment, that might have been an acceptable approach, but the damage had been done to our children and our family. We never returned to that counselor and instead, enrolled our whole family in a different counseling service. Eventually, we found someone who understood Sam's rebellion and helped us develop a more consistent plan to deal with his behaviors.

But by this time, we were adrift and needed some respite from the strains of childrearing.

Into the wilderness

Our family troubles were intensifying, and we were getting desperate. In middle school, Sam was suspended from one school, expelled from another, and refused admission to a third. Something had to change. Counseling was a complete failure and the Bible Camp had closed its doors to Rachel's participation in a camp for teenage girls. We were running out of places to turn before we completely lost control of our family.

I didn't know where to turn for help but reasoned that getting Sam back on the right path would help us deal with the growing problems in the family. Maybe a military school or some similar no-nonsense discipline setting would be the answer we were looking for. At least, it would provide a place to keep Sam safe. When I found one about one hundred miles away, we scheduled a tour.

Finding directions without a map was something I had always been proud of, and I wanted to impress Diane that I still had that skill. It's hard to carry on much of a conversation while driving a reluctant kid off to look at a boarding school. I consoled myself that we were making great time and would arrive in plenty of time for the tour. Diane and I managed to talk about how this trip to the military school might be the turn-around we were looking for. And it was a turn around. When I stopped for gas, I realized I had indeed made the trip in record time, only to the wrong city. We turned around and got to the military academy after most of the open house was completed. Was this a reflection of my breakneck pace of life and parenting, making great time, just ending up at the wrong destination? In the end, our late arrival didn't matter. The military school wasn't interested in trying to corral a child bent on bolting for freedom.

Finally, we found a place that agreed to take Sam, a wilderness program in the Utah desert where rebellious youth could get their lives in order. Sam agreed to our plan to enroll him in the desert program. Sam told me later that he was the only young person in his group that enrolled voluntarily. All the others in his group had been snatched out of their homes by hired transport guards in the middle of the night and transported to the program against their will. The flight to Utah was somber yet hopeful. Maybe this would be the breakthrough we all needed. Dropping Sam off with the program leader in Salt Lake City, a hasty goodbye, and a lonely and painful plane trip home all reinforced one theme: we had failed as parents.

How did this happen? Hadn't we been doing all the things involved parents were supposed to do? Didn't we follow all the rules? After almost two months in the Utah desert, the program felt Sam had made enough progress to be discharged. Or they could keep him for another several months for another $10-20,000 per month. Maybe it would help, but no guarantees. The wilderness program gave us temporary relief, but we were left with questions. How could we know if he had truly changed or if he just went along with the program for the experience? Would we ever see the end of his rebellious behavior? It wouldn't take long to find out. Two months in the wilderness weren't enough to overcome years of rebellious thinking.

As if we didn't feel enough guilt and shame at home, we felt an almost chronic sense of judgment from the people around us, people whose children never acted out, misbehaved, or did anything else that would be considered unacceptable. At least that's the impression we were given. Once, one of our kids had invited a friend to join us on a camping trip. Something went on between them the first night, kid stuff we thought. To our amazement, the friend's parents showed up at our campsite early the next morning to retrieve their child. No advance notice, no questions asked, no explanation offered. Maybe they felt they had to rescue their child, but from what? Struggling parents have enough difficulties to deal with. Had we known the basis for this unspoken criticism, we might have been able to benefit. Instead, we watched them drive away, we had been judged and found wanting.

Our sense of embarrassment increased with the worsening acts of rebellion. Having your kids steal from the collection plate isn't something they teach about in Sunday School. Sadness and shame, self-doubt and a sense of failure became our constant tormentors. We had long earlier abandoned our dreams of having a normal family. My brother Mark helped us navigate the school expulsions and ever-increasing legal issues (mostly related to drug use) piling up for the two rebellious children. Otherwise, we felt alone and isolated among our family and friends. I could identify with the lepers in the Bible calling out "Unclean, Unclean!" so others could keep their distance.

We dreaded receiving the self-congratulatory Christmas letters from friends and family with their endless lists of positive experiences and ever-increasing accomplishments of well-behaved children. What did we have to share? How would we have wanted others to respond?

Our faith in ourselves had been shaken. We had done everything we could imagine to develop and nurture our children, yet our approach just wasn't working. The stress was continual and increasing. And little did we realize, our problems were only going to get worse.

One by one, my illusions about parenting were being broken down, then shattered altogether. My whole life had been about trying to look good and having the right answers, but not this time. Whatever background I had from my family life, pediatric training, and Bible reading just couldn't solve the problems my family was experiencing. I simply didn't have any answers. Sam had taken rebellion to levels beyond anything we had ever imagined. Our rules weren't enough to prevent or even slow him down. He had presented us with one challenge after another. He was denied admission to one school after acting out on the school tour and expelled from another for selling marijuana. When we discovered a large quantity of marijuana stockpiled in our home, we notified the police. Our private lives had already been scrutinized by the counselors. Next, our home would be searched as well. I followed the police around the house dreading what else they might find.

Behind Bars and Plexiglass

It broke our hearts to know that in selling pot, our son was harming the lives of so many others. We just didn't know how to get him to stop. Sam had previously been arrested for stealing and spent time in a work-release jail setting. Waiting to pick him up, I observed the succession of inmates being released for the day, embarrassed that my son was now one of them. We hoped the time in jail would help Sam change his ways. It didn't turn out that way. Somewhere along the way, unknown to us, Sam picked up a firearm. While visiting a friend's house, an argument broke out between Sam and another person while the friend looked on. Sam pulled his gun and, in the scuffle, accidentally shot his friend in the leg. Sam spent almost a year in jail for that. No work-release this time. Jail was for serious offenders, the last stop before prison.

There's no way to capture the emotional experience of visiting your son in jail. It starts with making sure you keep quiet about it.

"What are you doing this weekend? Playing golf I suppose or maybe spending time at the cottage?"

"Oh, just spending time with family." End of discussion.

Everything about the jail, the narrow windows, surveillance cameras and warning signs is carefully designed to make it clear to visitors who is in charge. It started with the restricted visiting times, which certainly do not take into account that the visitors might have jobs or other responsibilities. The lobby resembled an old airport waiting area with hard plastic chairs and dirty floor but without the music. Maybe this is where their discarded furniture ends up. Unlike at the airport, though, nobody in this lounge is here because they really want to be. There are no excited conversations here, only subdued talk lest anyone overhear. No one wears a colorful travel outfit or carries souvenirs from their trip. There aren't any posters beckoning the traveler to far-off places, just warning signs: no eating or drinking, no music or loud talking. Few people make eye contact or attempt to meet others in the waiting room. After all, what do you have in common with them? What would you say to them as you secretly wonder what crime their loved one or friend had committed? The subdued visitors wait to be interrogated by the cold guards. Do they take a class on how to avoid having a friendly face?

The guards check to see if your name is on the approved visitor list. Do they have any sense of how hard this is? Does it even matter to them that the visitors aren't responsible for the choices the inmates have made. Or do they think the visitors are somehow responsible and should suffer a little too.

"Sorry, looks like you're not on the list. Try again another time. Next in line."

The visitor is continually reminded of their complete powerlessness. The guards and staff are protected by bulletproof glass, locked doors, and armed reinforcements. And they have guns. The visitor enters and empties their pockets and pride. After passing through another screening and metal detector, we're finally directed to Cellblock 3 to wait until our son is brought in.

Seeing Sam in jailhouse orange, talking to him over a phone through a plexiglass window, what does a parent say? How's it going? How's the food? How do you spend your day? Anything we can get you? Of course, there's nothing we can get him other than putting a few dollars in his jail account for snacks. (We had sent him a Bible, but it didn't get much use.) I hesitated to ask about any friends he might have made. I hoped he wasn't making friends in jail. I longed to hear something that suggested life-changing insight in our son, like in the movies.

Time's up. Sam is ushered back into his cell block, and we're directed back to the long corridor to the lobby. On the way, our personal belongings are returned to us. Our pride gets left behind. Finally, we exit through another set of locked doors, eyed over with more suspicious looks from the guards. The lobby is now empty, and the room will be quiet until the arrival of the next group of hurting and broken loved ones.

Back in the parking lot, still under surveillance, we saw ourselves as utter failures as parents. What can we say to each other that's positive? Only twenty-seven more weeks to go until Sam gets out, or was it twenty-eight?

Life seemed to settle down for a while after Sam was released from jail until our family situation took another turn for the worse. Within a several month period, my mom and Diane's dad both died after short illnesses. We would no longer benefit from the wisdom and support of two of the steadiest and most influential persons in our lives.

About a year after he was released from jail, Sam, now twenty years old, was living in a duplex with a friend. He worked a job in direct sales (of legal products) and planned to attend business school. When Sam visited us on Mother's Day, we had a conversation I distinctly recall about his living situation. Sam felt that his current housing was risky, and he wanted to know if he could move home. We had discussed this before and I assured Sam that we always had an open door for him. But he had to agree to abide by a couple of nonnegotiable rules meant to protect his younger sister and brother. He would have to agree not to sell drugs or keep supplies of drugs around our house. Sam told me he couldn't do that.

During our conversation, I observed that Sam had grown up in a strongly Christian home with both parents present. He had all the opportunities that life in America could afford, yet he chose to rebel and follow his own path. How, I asked, could a person have all those advantages and not be held accountable at some point? I believed God would get his attention one way. I hoped and prayed he would make changes before it was too late. Sam listened, but in the end, Sam went back to the duplex. I had no idea how much danger he was in.

Chapter 14

Left for Dead

I had only heard about you but now, I have seen you with my own eyes.

Job 42:5 (NLT)

Paralyzed

The day began on a festive note with Rachel's bridal shower luncheon. The wedding date was only three weeks away. We were also celebrating Diane's birthday. Typically each of our kids call or visit on our birthdays and other big events. One after another, our children called Diane with birthday wishes, each of them, except Sam. This was distinctly unusual for even with his ongoing struggles, Sam always stayed in touch..

I started the day at the Cellcom half marathon check-in activity, picking up my T-shirt and race packet for the following morning's race. Diane spent much of the afternoon helping a friend cook for her son's graduation party. Earlier in the day, we received a call from the police inquiring about Sam's whereabouts. We hadn't heard from him but checked with his work and found he hadn't come in that day, another unusual occurrence for someone as conscientious as Sam. In the early evening, the police called back to tell us they had found Sam's burned up van in a remote wooded area. Could we help locate him?

We checked with each of our kids to see if they had any information. Tony had been shooting pool with Sam the night before but they finished early. Sam wanted to get a good night's rest before working the next morning. Rachel and her fiancé Justin agreed to go over to Sam's duplex to see if they could figure out what was going on. When they arrived, they found the front door ajar and Sam semi-conscious on his bed, bleeding from his neck, unable to move. They called 911 and waited for help to arrive. The EMTs and police were on the scene in a matter of minutes.

It was a blur of activity after that. The EMTs stabilized Sam and transported him to the nearby Aurora Hospital. The police searched the home and found Sam's roommate dead in the basement, shot in the back of the head, execution style. They first questioned Rachel and Justin at the duplex and then took them to the police station for further interrogation. We rushed to meet Sam at the Emergency Department full of anxious questions. Sam had lost a lot of blood and was unable to breathe effectively due to the gunshot. The bullet grazed the underside of his jaw and went through the spinal cord, causing instant paralysis below the C4-5 level. Had the bullet path been even one or two millimeters in any direction, Sam almost certainly would have bled to death or died from respiratory failure.

The hospital is supposed to be a safe place for the patient and family but that wasn't how things were for us. Someone informed us that there was going to be another attempt on Sam's life in the hospital. We needed to take precautions. We started to learn of the details of the shootings and reconstruct the crime after the police apprehended the assailant. After a dispute about some drug dealings, he had murdered Sam's roommate and then attempted to steal Sam's van to flee.

When Sam regained the ability to speak, he told us the rest of the story and how he woke up to find the assailant in the process of stealing the keys to his van. When Sam tried to stop him, he shot Sam almost point blank with a comment to the effect of, "Say goodbye to your face." As much as it could be possible, justice ended up being served. For the murder and attempted murder, the killer received a life sentence in prison without possibility of parole.

A couple of weeks after his injury, Sam was transported by helicopter to the regional medical center in Milwaukee for ongoing care. As the flight nurses strapped him onto the stretcher, I thought of how many times I myself had been on such a transport team in my training. I had never given much thought to what that must have been like for the anxious parents who stood by helplessly watching us. Now I was the one watching, afraid, powerless.

This was the start of our year-long odyssey from hospital to treatment center to residential care facilities, each time hoping that Sam might show some return of muscle function. The smallest hint of improvement, a little more strength in his left hand, some movement in the shoulder, raised our hopes, only there would be no additional recovery. Sam would never regain the physical abilities he had lost. Even worse, he would continuously suffer from chronic pain. Thankfully, his mind remained as sharp as ever.

Several episodes in the hospital and rehabilitation centers highlighted how little doctors sometimes listen to their patients. In one hospital, Sam was supposed to begin physical therapy, but was groggy and didn't seem to show much interest in the rehab program. The doctor asserted that it was because Sam was lazy and not motivated to help out with his own recovery. Sam was in a lot of pain at the time for which he was receiving strong narcotics. I suggested to the staff that perhaps Sam was sedated from all the pain medication. I had never known him to be lazy in his entire life.

The medical team dismissed what I had to say. Though they were medical school faculty, I knew my son better than they did. The next day, Sam woke up and was soon back to his old self. Overnight, the staff had administered Narcan, a medication that reverses the harmful effects of the narcotics he was receiving. They assured me that their choice of treatment had nothing to do with my suggestion. They had figured that out themselves.

Once he was out of the crisis stage, Sam was transferred to the Courage Center, a rehabilitation facility in Minneapolis. There we learned firsthand of the fate of many persons with spinal cord injuries and what life could look like for them. Sam's roommate was a man with quadriplegia who never had any visitors. Like many with similar injuries, he had been deserted by his family and friends apart from holiday visits. Our family resolved to never abandon Sam.

We met many others with spinal cord injuries who were lonely, bitter, and depressed, but we felt that our involvement would prevent that outcome for Sam. One day, this delusion was broken when we got a call from Sam. He told us that he had managed to drive his power wheelchair off the grounds of the Courage Center. He was near a busy roadway and was considering driving his chair into oncoming traffic. Thankfully, we were able to talk him down and make arrangements for the staff to bring him back to safety. Another time, we found him using what little upper body strength he had to try to get a hold of a knife to harm himself. Another time, he planned to drown himself by driving his chair into a retention pond.

Thanksgiving Dinner in the ICU

Give thanks in all circumstances.

1 Thessalonians 5:18 (ESV)

Holiday traditions and meals hold our family together in difficult times. It was the day before Thanksgiving and Diane was visiting Sam at the Courage Center. I was planning to join them the next day with a dinner prepared by our friends. We had eaten too many holiday meals in hospital cafeterias over my years of medical school, training, and practice, always the same food and the same forced effort to celebrate surrounded by anxious visitors and busy hospital staff. We wanted Sam to have family around him and enjoy home cooking this first holiday after the shooting.

Late in the afternoon, Diane called to tell me Sam had developed sepsis and had been admitted to the ICU at a nearby hospital. He had been hospitalized many times, so I was used to these kinds of calls. This time was different. A nurse came on the line and advised me Sam was conscious and stable but I shouldn't delay coming. "Your son might not make it through the night. Tomorrow afternoon may be too late." Having worked all day in the clinic, it didn't seem safe for me to drive late that night. But I had to get to see Sam. Diane contacted our volunteer cooks who readied the food for the drive while I got a few hours of sleep before the five hour drive. Sam's condition stabilized so I could bring the food up the next day.

How does one get a Thanksgiving meal into the ICU waiting room without getting stopped by security? Time to improvise. We loaded the food into a wheelchair and covered it with a blanket. As we wheeled the "patient" into the lobby, I commented that it was time to get this turkey back into the hospital. The security guards nodded, probably aware of what we were up to, but they graciously allowed us to pass.

A palpable tension fills an ICU waiting room, with its hospital smell and sterile furniture and anxious, preoccupied visitors, strangers yet with something in common. The TV does most of the talking and drowns out the subdued conversations, reminiscent of the visitors' area at the jail where we once visited Sam for a different holiday.

Before we could eat, a nurse in scrubs entered the room. Everyone looked up with a mixture of hope and dread. Conversations stopped, replaced by unspoken questions. Is there some news? Has something happened to my loved one?

Diane and I were relieved when someone else was summoned to talk privately. Our hearts went out to them; we feared the nurse could be coming for us next. How many times had I walked into a waiting room as the doctor to deliver bad news? Now I was on the receiving end. Roles reversed.

As we set out the food, the room fills with comforting aromas. Each of our friends must have selected their favorite recipe. One prepared the turkey and stuffing, others made side dishes, sweet potatoes, green bean casserole, cranberries, and homemade rolls. Then there were the pies! We had everything typically associated with a traditional Thanksgiving feast. Well almost everything. Our son was clinging to life in the ICU.

I looked around at the other visitors. Where were they going to celebrate their Thanksgiving? In the cafeteria? Huddled around a vending machine? I invited them to join us. They politely declined. "No thanks, not hungry." But their looks said something else. Time for a different approach. I made up a platter of turkey sandwiches and set them out on a coffee table. Before long, the children in the waiting room sought their parents' permission and cautiously began to sample our offerings. Parents followed right behind. Soon it was time to prepare another platter, pass around the sides and serve up the pies.

Over dinner, we shared our stories and asked about how each other's loved one was doing. One man asked to borrow the Bible I was reading. I shared how it was faith in God that got our family through our troubles. Years later, I came across the man's thank you note tucked in the Bible, a reminder of the time we shared more than a meal in the ICU waiting room.

Our Thanksgiving dinner in the ICU nourished more than our bodies. Extending hospitality to strangers took our minds off our own suffering. We brought the food, our new friends brought us encouragement and understanding. When Sam was transferred out of the ICU, we learned that ours was one of the few families at that Thanksgiving dinner whose loved one survived their stay in the ICU.

Several days later, I tried to stay overnight with Sam. He was still in serious condition, but at least he was in a regular room. I was reluctant to leave him. I've never done well sleeping in a chair, so after the nurses made their rounds, I tried to rest on the cold marble floor near his bed. I had spent countless nights in on-call rooms over my career and even lived in a hospital for a month during medical school. On my mission trips abroad, I saw parents sleeping under the cribs in the pediatric ward helping to provide care for their children. Now I was one of those parents sleeping on the floor, keeping a vigil over their child.

Suddenly, alarms sounded, and the dark room was full of doctors and nurses. Sam's heart had stopped! Airway, breathing, circulation!

Activity everywhere. I was told to leave the room. I couldn't do anything to help Sam at this point, just stay out of the way. Would this be the end? Thankfully, Sam quickly responded to the emergency treatment.

How does life go on when you're in the midst of this type of trauma? Diane was our family's primary support for Sam and spent many weeks and weekends visiting him in Minneapolis. She often took Peter, age twelve, along for the visits, home schooling him in the process. Our other kids kept busy with school and work. They seemed to be doing well as far as I could tell, though I never realized how much the stress affected them.

I'm not sure my response to the trauma was the best. I returned to work in my solo allergy practice, afraid to find out what might happen from a financial standpoint if I had dropped out of practice for a while. Work also helped me maintain some stability in my own thinking by doing the things I knew best.

It's remarkable how a person can compartmentalize their thinking and somehow function in times of such great trauma and stress. Spouse, children, work, and finances all require continual attention. Unlike algebra, though, there's no perfect solution to the variables in this equation. My patients continued to do well throughout this time, and, for this, I'm quite thankful. Unfortunately, the same can't be said for my family. We had each suffered in different ways, though we were never able to acknowledge it or talk about it. By the end of the first couple of years after the injury, we entered the long process of caring for our loved one with quadriplegia, a journey that will continue for the rest of our lives.

My spiritual beliefs have told me that good can certainly come out of suffering. Living through Sam's paralysis and its effect on our family helped me empathize with my own patients. They too suffer from serious problems. Their concerns may not be as dramatic as mine, but they are just as valid and important. They deserve just as much attention as anything going on in my life.This deeper connection with the lives of others contributed to my interest in reflective writing and narrative medicine.

It has been hard to resist getting consumed by these life-altering traumas and surrender to the tendency to withdraw from life and all its demands. My habit of regular exposure to the Scriptures gave me strength to carry on. I struggled to find the balance between supporting my family and being strengthened through contact with others. I chose to continue to serve at church; teaching God's Word to others had always given me a purpose. Now, continuing to teach helped me survive.

Unfortunately, there was a downside to the way our family tried to recover from Sam's injuries. Apart from the time I was fired, I've never been good at seeking counseling. When we sought help with our rebellious children, counseling only seemed to make matters worse. But this time our needs were different. Our family needed someone to talk to, someone we could trust to help us make sense of our different emotions and our individual responses to Sam's injuries. We never sought this kind of help, too busy trying to survive. Sadly, it would take years for us to really know how Sam's condition has affected each of us differently..

Failed by the system

Sam's injury and its aftermath made me acutely aware of some of the worst features of our contemporary American medical system. The paradoxes and shortcomings were obvious. The acute care Sam received was consistently fabulous, demonstrating the skill and expertise of his medical team. I wish I could say the same about his chronic care. I had always seen the medical system from the standpoint of its many successes. As a physician, I was in a position of authority. People listened to my voice and followed my lead. As a parent, the experience was quite different.

My role had always been to provide for others, not to admit that I needed their help. The stress of severe trauma, became my lesson in humility, and taught me to see my own patients in a different, more understanding way.

In the hospital, each floor unit had its own social workers and case managers to oversee the details of Sam's care and placement. Their job was to ensure that the correct follow-along care would be provided. However, in a larger hospital, the patient is frequently moved from one floor to another based on the level of care needed. This meant a switch from one social worker or case manager to another. With each transfer, a whole new team would have to learn the complexities of Sam's care. More records to review, more questions to be repeated. The inefficiencies were glaring. While they took time to learn about Sam, there seemed to be little interest in trying to understand and support his family. Never mind that we were the ones who would be caring for him for the long term.

In the fifteen years since the shooting, Sam has averaged one surgery per year for the complications of his paralysis. It's difficult to see him suffering from chronic pain, especially knowing he's tried so many different treatments without success. I don't know how many times I left his apartment in tears as I considered just how much suffering he has endured. Eventually, his doctors have essentially said they have nothing more to offer him.

When Sam's paralysis became a permanent part of our lives, we needed to make a choice. Would we consider ourselves victims of the tragic circumstances we were enduring? Is this what will define us from now on? In earlier times of loss, I had chosen to do my best to conquer setbacks, and this time would be no different.

Our faith was sorely tested through all these family trials, but at each step of the way, it was strengthened as well. When we felt abandoned by those around us, we could trust that God would never leave us. When we felt judged by others, we could rely on the scripture that reminds us that there's no condemnation for those who love God. We had seen too many examples of how God was at work in our lives. He provided a place for us to stay when Sam was in the hospital in Milwaukee and another home for us to stay at when he was in Minnesota. Sam pulled through all the crises, surgeries, and even a cardiac arrest and has come through this as a different person. Another act of God.

Looking for a fallout shelter

As children, we were constantly reminded that our country was in grave peril of a nuclear war. Everyone was instructed to know where to go for protection should that occur. Fallout shelters were developed around the country, from public buildings to private homes, like my sisters storing up supplies in a bedroom closet in the event of an attack. I would have liked a shelter from the nuclear storm that had hit our family but there was no way to escape or hide. I had tried to store up supplies of a different sort but they didn't protect me.

There's no easy way to describe how an event like this can shape the lives of an entire family. With the succession of hospitals and treatment centers, the nights and weeks away from home, and the constant sense of dread about Sam's condition, our other children were left adrift at times.

Diane and I had tried to model a stable, healthy marriage for our children, but we couldn't ensure this result for them. Rachel, Tony, and Peter had each gotten married since Sam's injury, Rachel barely two weeks after the shooting. I failed to anticipate the challenges our married kids were going to face and eventually, all three of them divorced. Perhaps there might have been different outcomes if I had spoken out sooner when I first saw problems developing. Instead, not wanting to alienate anyone, I reverted to my non-confrontational middle child approach from childhood. Should any of them remarry, I'll be much more vigilant and forthright with them.

A pilgrimage yields some answers

"Now serving breakfast in the dining car!" The cheerful, inviting comment rang out through our train car, awakening us as Peter and I crossed the Northern Plains on the Amtrak Empire Builder. The rhythmic cadence (iambic pentameter) still stands out as our secret knock, a reminder of his eighth grade homeschool graduation trip to the Dakotas. Three years had passed since Sam's shooting and we planned to retrace some of the steps of the Lewis and Clark Expedition and make a side trip to my birthplace. I wanted to show Peter the magical place where my family had lived so many years earlier. More than that, I wanted to see my birthplace again and try to get a better understanding of how life in that small town could have had such an impact on our family. I wasn't sure I would meet anyone who even remembered us.

These forays into northern South Dakota became part of the legacy my siblings and I shared. Even the ones who had never lived there shared this homing instinct. Like pilgrims following the path of some holy person, we were in search of a miracle of sorts, an insight into how our family life was influenced by our life on the northern plains. After each visit, we would relate stories of the people and places we encountered to the rest of the family. Diane and I stopped there on our honeymoon where we met some of Dad's former patients and heard their stories of the care they had received from Dad years earlier.

Peter and I made our pilgrimage more than fifty years after our family had moved back to Wisconsin. Though our family hadn't stayed in touch with anyone in McLaughlin, on visits to the Senior Center we met several of Dad's former patients and their descendants. They still remembered the doctor with the large family and told of Dad's legendary service in their community. Appreciative patients shared memories of winter house calls in blizzard conditions and emergency surgeries and how they often paid their bills with chickens and produce.

I began to wonder what kind of care would a doctor have to provide for people to remember him sixty years later. How much time away from home would that kind of care require? I once heard it said that "The patient's meat is the doctor's poison." Patients want their physician with the three A's: Able to solve complex problems; Approachable in any situation; Available at all times. Dad was all these and more, ever ready to sacrifice personal needs for the patient's welfare. Wasn't I doing the same myself, often leaving my family behind as I pursued my own dreams? Maybe I was more like my dad than I realized or wanted to admit.

Standing in front of our old house, I thought back to one of the stories we still share about life in McLaughlin. One day, Dad came home from the clinic for lunch and found a group of children playing in the front yard. As it has been related to me, he told the children they should be getting home when one of my siblings responded, "But Dad, we live here!" Humorous, I thought, until I questioned whether I had made myself too busy and preoccupied to recognize my own children.

I never realized how hard moving could be on a family. It all sounds so romantic, new places, new friends, new opportunities. Then reality crashes the party. This was my mother's first move away from her supportive family. And our family kept growing, adding five more children in five years. It was up to Mom to manage the household while Dad and his partner ran the clinic and covered the local hospital.

And then there was Susie's illness. In my years of medical training, I had worked at regional referral hospitals caring for children who had traveled long distances for care. Hundreds of miles from home, their families anxiously waited for any positive news about their child. Standing there in that little South Dakota town, I could now imagine what it must have been like for my parents as they desperately prayed for the recovery that never came.

Following Susie's death, my mom was heartbroken. Years later, she spoke with unmistakable sadness as she described the lonely winter drive back to Wisconsin for the funeral. Grieving parents and confused children rode in the car; Dad's brother Reggie accompanied Susie's casket on the train. As a family, we never talked about how hard it was to lose a child or how lonely it was to be so far from home. We never discussed how powerless Dad must have felt, the bright and capable physician who could care for so many others but was unable to save his own daughter. I was left to wonder if this is what spurred Dad's aggressive treatment of my sore throat that school morning years ago.

The pilgrimage to my birthplace turned out to be more than another homeschool field trip for Peter. It changed my understanding of how the years in South Dakota had shaped our family. The hospital is closed now, and the town looks tired and run down, anything but magical. But the legacy of the town that never exceeded 1000 residents continues to impact me and my siblings, as well as our own children and grandchildren.

PART FIVE

FAITH PREVAILS

Chapter 15

A Practice of my Own

For I know the plans I have for you, declares the Lord, plans to prosper you and not to harm you, plans to give you hope and a future.

Jeremiah 29:11 (NIV)

By the end of a career in medicine, a physician could log as many as 100,000 patient visits or more. It wouldn't be possible to tell about each visit, but some patients stand out. For me, these were ones who touched me in an emotional way or taught me something about myself. Their lives may have been changed through the care they received, but mine was too.

Many doctors ask the question, "What's the matter?" They should also be asking the patient, "What matters most?" This one question transformed my medical practice by allowing me to get to the heart of whatever was most important for each patient. For a nurse with asthma, what mattered most was that she be able to play with her children in the front yard without suffering an asthma attack. For an older adult, what mattered most was to be able to breathe without difficulty even if it meant taking low doses of Prednisone, a potent drug with many possible side effects. For children, what mattered most might be as simple as being able to sleep at night so they could stay awake during the day at school. Parents had dreams for their young children; adult children expressed different dreams for their elderly parents. My joy came from helping each of them achieve what they longed for.

Allergy practice had many similarities with studying the Bible. Both required asking a lot of questions and paying close attention to the answers, as well as considering the setting of events and the context in which they occurred.

Even while Sam was recovering from his injuries, I needed to continue seeing patients. While it was difficult to be away from him, my work helped me maintain my focus on my calling to be a doctor. The following vignettes tell of some of the remarkable people who shaped my thinking about patient care over my three decades in practice. They provides a glimpse into some of the patients and families who were to become my teachers:

"She's going to die, just like me"

It started with an allergy consultation at the hospital for a repeated ICU admission for a preteen girl. Nothing from the history explained the severity and poor control of her asthma but something was seriously wrong. I hadn't figured it out the first time we met. I may not get another chance. Asthma can be fatal. Searching for a clue to the child's life-threatening condition, I asked her mother,

"What do you think is going to happen to your daughter as a result of her asthma?"

She replied without any trace of emotion, "Oh, she's going to die from her asthma."

"Why do you say that?"

"Well, that's what's going to happen to me."

By her late twenties, this mother was already seeking disability status for her own breathing troubles. Since the child's grandfather also suffered from severe asthma, the family had developed a fatalistic attitude toward the child's prospects. Treating the patient required helping her family recognize that things didn't have to turn out that way. There was hope that their child could live a normal life. With this new understanding, the patient and her family became active participants in developing an asthma management strategy. The last I heard, this young girl had graduated from college and the severe asthma was no longer such a problem.

When everybody else has given up

Having faith in your patient's ability to succeed is crucial when dealing with emotion-laden problems. Richard, a high school student, was in danger of dropping out of school. His poor grades and frequent absences were considered signs of his lack of motivation. His asthma was under poor control and physical activities were limited. Talking with him revealed his sense of hopelessness. For him, asthma care would require far more than selection of the right medications.

Working together, he and I developed a plan starting with getting his asthma and allergies under control. This helped him regain his self-respect and sense of control over his life. Next, we had to address the school's concerns. His guidance counselor was skeptical about his prospects for improvement. She happened to be a patient of mine as well, and I was able to personally advocate for this young man's educational program. Our mutual efforts were a success. He eventually went on to become a computer programmer.

"Why should I put down the magazine?"

The patients who touched me most deeply were those who were disadvantaged in some way. For some, it was lack of financial resources or difficult living circumstances. For others, it was the consequences of the poor choices they had made. Most touching of all were the ones who had been treated badly by the medical system.

A mother sat disinterestedly as I examined her son. She was engrossed in a magazine while I tried to evaluate the child's asthma. She never looked up as we talked but said she agreed with my recommended plan of action. On the follow up visit, out came the magazine once again. The patient had improved but we needed to make some adjustments in medications. Again I wondered if his mother was even listening? How could I get her attention without offending her to ensure that she understood our treatment plan? I shared my concern and was shocked by her response.

"Why shouldn't I read a magazine? Where we come from, nobody cares about us at the doctor's office."

"Well," I replied, "in this office we do care about you. Give us a chance to prove it."

This child went on to do well with his asthma. He and his mother taught me that there are many reasons for a patient's behavior that may have nothing to do with me or my clinic. How sad to realize that some patients suffer at the hands of the healthcare system. I resolved to do my best to avoid that in my patients.

At the funeral home

I attended several funerals of patients over the years as my way of showing support for their families. On some occasions, failure to take prescribed asthma medication contributed to their death. A former patient had apparently died from an asthma attack, and I wanted to express my condolences to her family. In medical school, we had been trained to approach patients without establishing any type of emotional attachment. While this might protect both the doctor and patient from any number of problems, I found it difficult to provide care for people without ever really knowing them. What obstacles prevented patients from achieving the best medical care? What kept them from following advice or taking their medications? Sometimes, I felt powerless watching a patient make choices that would eventually lead to severe, even fatal, consequences. Yet I couldn't stop them. I couldn't force them to quit smoking or take regularly prescribed medications or show up for scheduled follow up visits.

Back to Asthma Camp

Patient evaluations aren't limited to the history and physical exam. The patient's physical and social environment and the patient's capabilities must also be considered. For me to accomplish this meant sponsoring a series of asthma camps for children and their parents. In a typical asthma camp, our team taught asthma self-care to asthmatic children. The camp was staffed by nurses, respiratory therapists, pharmacists, and an occupational therapist, as well as numerous healthcare students. For parents, we conducted information sessions and support groups.

The impact of asthma on a child's self-image became apparent to me at our first asthma camp. One of the children went missing right after being checked in. We hurriedly searched the area only to find the missing child in the car with his mother. He was taking a few puffs of his bronchodilator inhaler. "Why are you out here in the car?"

"I needed to take my inhaler and I didn't want anyone else to know that I had asthma."

How remarkable! A child enrolled in a camp where all the children had asthma didn't want the other campers to know that he had asthma. His mother waited in the parking lot to make sure that everything was okay, even though her child was surrounded by medical personnel. This was another transforming experience, learning firsthand the impact asthma was having on patients and their families.

Following Dad to the tribal clinic

Taking medical care out into the community also involved returning to my role as a consultant to the Oneida Community Health Center on Green Bay's west side. When I was growing up, the Native American people in our area suffered greatly from discrimination, poverty, unemployment, and alcohol abuse. The advent of gaming on tribal lands provided the tribe with a steady source of revenue which they used to provide needed services for their members.

The traditional monthly consultant clinic would have a specialist to see as many patients as possible, one patient at a time. My model was going to be different, patterned after my Air Force experience with the visiting allergist. I would use each clinic session to see patients and then train the staff to apply the same level of care for the rest of the month. The staff and patients at the Health Center taught me about cultural and religious practices including natural remedies and sweat lodges, some which might provoke asthmatic reactions.

Growing up, I never had any direct contact with Native Americans. All my knowledge was based on portrayals in the media. As I conducted my clinics, I began to see them as part of a community and hear them share their hopes and dreams.

The Oneida tribe also invited us to use their ropes course for an asthma camp. Following the asthma education time, the campers donned safety harnesses and climbed up to the high elements. At first fearful, then tentative, finally emboldened, they took turns traversing the highest level trusting a staff member or another camper to belay them for safety. What a perfect image of the trust and teamwork needed to provide the best medical care.

"I know we're not at the clinic but..."

Patients also had an impact on me outside the clinic and hospital where unexpected questions arose. Should I acknowledge our professional relationship while out socially? Wouldn't this violate principles of confidentiality? There were many occasions when I would get into a conversation with a friend and my wife would be amazed that I had been providing care for them for some time. I was always careful to maintain my patients' privacy but sometimes they would approach me in public. As their physician, I really couldn't ignore them or their questions. I've looked at many skin rashes in the lobby at church as patients lifted up their shirts or stuck out an arm or leg for me to examine.

On one occasion, Diane and I were on a ferry ride across Lake Michigan when a woman approached us on the deck. "Doctor Warpinski," she asked, "if I fell overboard would you jump over the railing to save me?" My wife later told me she was perplexed that a complete stranger would ask such a question. Shouldn't the woman's own husband jump into the lake to save her? Put on the spot, I replied that I would try to get help for her as quickly as I could but that if I tried to save her, we would both likely drown.

What matters most?

Ricardo was a ten-year-old boy with asthma who was seen for an initial visit. His history of respiratory symptoms seemed fairly straightforward. His history physical exam and breathing tests supported the diagnosis of asthma, like so many other patients I'd seen. It looked like a pretty straightforward case: prescribe asthma medications to get control of the symptoms, encourage exercise and schedule a follow-up visit. These measures would be considered adequate for our first encounter, but a merely adequate visit wasn't what this boy really needed.

I had been reading about a new subject called Narrative Medicine and decided to give it a try. This meant I would need to pay closer attention to some of the details of the visit I might have otherwise overlooked: the clothing worn, specific words used, emotions, and facial expressions. I started to see the young boy and his mother differently. I was confident that I had the answers they needed until I asked mother the question that changed my practice from that time on:

"What matters most to you about your son's health? What would you like him to be able to do if he didn't have asthma?"

Mother broke down in tears. "I just want him to be able to play outside."

I learned that Ricardo wasn't allowed to play outside because of his asthma. Instead, he had to watch his friends play soccer outside while he was sheltered in the safety of his home. Being restricted like that was bad enough, but that wasn't the whole reason for mother's distress. Her older son played semi-professional soccer in Mexico and Ricardo dreamed of doing the same. This was the crucial missing information that told me just how severely this boy's asthma was affecting him.

With this shared understanding of what motivated this patient and his family, we developed a treatment plan together. Within a couple of years, Ricardo moved to Mexico to join his brother. Definitely, this was a successful outcome for all of us. Asking the right questions and taking time to listen to the answers, the foundational practices of narrative medicine, had made all the difference.

A short while after Ricardo's initial visit, I attended an education workshop that explained how writing out patient narratives could change the way the doctor sees the patient and family. The speaker instructed us to begin the process by recording as many details as possible. I didn't realize it at the time, but she was really making a case for being "all there" during the patient encounter, basically putting mindfulness in action. I thought back to Ricardo with his engaging smile. I pictured him sitting on the exam table, well groomed, wearing a polo shirt with broad blue and white horizontal stripes.

His mother wore a red print pattern dress, her dark brown hair pulled back. With her limited English language skills, she and I talked about her concerns for her son who filled in occasional words as needed. (This was a time when interpreters weren't readily available for clinic visits. Now, having a nonfamily member interpreter is considered a patient's right.)

Composing this narrative account of our visit produced an immediate sense of deeper connection with Ricardo and his mother. When I shared my writing with them at their next visit, mother expressed her appreciation for the time and effort that went into truly seeing her and her son. This is the same response I receive from others who are touched that someone would try to capture their story.

Unsustainable life; set apart from others

Solo practice had served me and my patients well in terms of autonomy, control, and freedom to be myself in my work and pursue my dreams. I was able to support my family and see all of my children launched from our home. But the freedom of running my own practice for over twenty years was taking a toll.

Not only was I responsible for a large cohort of patients, I also had to manage the office hiring, policies, recruiting, and finances. The harder I tried to balance all of these responsibilities, the less my efforts were appreciated. I found myself constrained from helping employees in need lest I run afoul of some employment law, fearful of making some mistake.

Diane strongly encouraged me to consider selling my practice to a local hospital to escape these pressures. Fortunately, I had learned from my previous mistakes and listened to her advice. Diane's other concern at the time was that I might develop some health problem that would keep me from working. I'd be at risk of losing the practice and our income if I weren't able to keep seeing patients.

Unfortunately, in resolving these concerns, I violated the promise I had made to myself many years earlier. Selling my practice was supposed to free me from the uncertainties and burdens of independent practice. Instead, the loss of autonomy and control led to depression and increasing burnout.

Something had to change before my mental health compromised patient care. A several month long program on physician burnout had recently been started by the State Medical Society. Maybe this would show me where I needed to change so I could continue in practice. But the program emphasized something completely different. In most cases of physician burnout, the doctor isn't the main problem. The real issue is the work environment itself, something which doctors, myself included, were powerless to change.

Chapter 16

The Doctor Abroad

How beautiful on the mountains are the feet of those who bring good news.

Isaiah 52:7 (NIV)

Learning a better way to do missions

Few things reveal the depth of one's values better than their response to a healthy dose of failure. Ten years after the ill-advised trip to Hungary, while still in my independent practice days, a friend invited me to take time off from my clinic and travel with him to Trinidad. His mission organization had been asked to conduct public health clinics sponsored by local churches. The pastors viewed these clinics as a means to reach out to their respective rural communities. The Hungary trip had completely changed my approach to missions. Overseas trips would no longer be self-centered ventures that would leave my family behind. Diane and I agreed that she and our five children should be added to future mission teams whenever possible. Eventually, Diane joined me for several trips to Trinidad, Rachel came as an adult, Emily as a teenager and Peter at age eleven. What a difference this made compared to my prior self-centered approach to missions. The following vignettes give some idea of the way short term missions can be valuable experiences for all parties involved. Most of them took place while I was still in practice.

Medical care costs one day

Our public health clinics provided basic physical exams and diabetes screening. We answered health-related questions posed by the clinic attendees. Sometimes, a person wanted our opinion on the care they were receiving from their own doctor. Other times, it was quite clear that patients had little confidence in the government-provided care. One older woman came to the clinic without any medical concerns. She waited in line just to have her picture taken with an American doctor.

I asked one clinic attendee about the cost of medical care which was reportedly free. The response surprised me. "Medical care costs one day. Either you spend a day waiting in the "free" clinic or you pay a day's wages to be seen by a private doctor.

With only limited resources, we had to find creative ways to answer people's questions. When a young woman came to the clinic anxious about having diabetes, it was time to improvise. Blood sugar testing can help diagnose obvious cases of diabetes, but more sophisticated tests would be needed to determine a person's future risk for that condition. Back at home, we could do a glucose tolerance; here, we performed a "pineapple mango challenge." Eat several slices of pineapple, drink a couple glasses of mango juice and return in two hours for a blood sugar test. The results of our test helped us advise the concerned woman that her body didn't handle sugar as well as it needed to. Changes in her diet might help her avoid diabetes. She should be sure to follow up with her regular doctor as well.

The Trinidad trips were not only about the medical clinics. We devoted time to leadership development and teaching in the local churches and attended prayer meetings and other church activities. The team was lodged in a house down the road from our host church so we could walk to attend any services. Crowding eight or ten missionaries into a house without running water challenged us to maintain the right spiritual attitude (not to mention daily hygiene.)

One day we were stopped along the way to the church by a man who asked us to pray with him about a setback he had experienced in his life. Our team was going to be late for the scheduled church meeting if we stopped for long. We had to decide what to do. How ironic, I thought, that we might have to tell the man we were too busy to pray with him because we were on our way to a prayer meeting. We resolved the dilemma by briefly praying with the man and promising to come back the next day for a more extended discussion. The following morning, we learned that his wife had left him, and he wasn't sure what to do next. I could sense the anxiety coming from his unexpected loss of a loved one; I had felt that growing up.

Mission trips gave me opportunities to do things I would rarely be able to do at home. On one trip, a friend and I were guest speakers on a live call-in radio program. I fielded the first question: "What do you think about drinking horse urine to treat asthma?" Not the question I was expecting. Fortunately, I had studied topics like this with my interest in the history of medicine. In response to the caller, I was able to say with certainty that horse urine is not a recommended treatment for asthma, though many believed that in the past. We have more effective remedies now. Appreciating the historical approaches to medical treatment can lead to greater understanding of therapies used in other cultures.

While the clinics sounded good in theory, the entire effort was hampered by the lack of a unified vision between the local churches as to the purpose of these clinics. Even after a total of 10 trips, the clinics continued to suffer from a lack of consistency and follow up. Our trips had introduced over 100 team members to the mission field and we had served several thousand people in the clinics. Unfortunately, without any significant plan for bringing healthcare to the communities we attempted to serve, the entire clinic program eventually folded. The churches and the mission group moved on to other things. Very disappointing.

From all these trips, I learned that serving others is more complicated than simply addressing their perceived needs. Effective service must find the balance between providing immediate relief, promoting restoration of health and well-being, and pursuing long-term development and self-sufficiency. A dedicated local partner is essential.

I also learned that spirituality looks very different in developing countries, where new believers commonly spend up to a year being mentored by their churches. There is a much greater sense of God's active presence in the world with people talking freely of their miraculous experiences.

A unique teaching moment

When the Trinidad trips ended, I looked for other ways to fulfill my desire to serve on the mission field. CMDA sponsored a teaching trip to a former Soviet republic to teach at a medical school, make rounds at a rehabilitation center and provided encouragement to members of the local Christian medical community. I was now involved in medical education through my practice and wanted to see how doctors are trained in other countries. The trip taught me that some aspects of medical education acceptable in former Soviet countries would never be tolerated in the United States. Some clinical teachers limited what they taught their students so they wouldn't learn too much and take the teacher's patients. In some cases, a student with the right connections could reportedly obtain a medical degree without actually taking the needed courses and passing the licensing exams. Much of the training was lecture-based and the students were primarily encouraged to memorize lists of possible diagnoses associated with different signs and symptoms. Hands-on physical diagnosis skills and clinical reasoning received much less attention.

At the medical school, I was scheduled to deliver a lecture to senior physicians and students on pediatric food allergy. Less than half an hour before the talk was to begin, a call came from the Director's office summoning me to do a consultation on the child of one of the staff members. To refuse such a request would be a serious breach of protocol, and the rest of the day's packed schedule wouldn't allow the time needed for this. Time to improvise. I invited the mother and her son to join me in the lecture hall. Weaving the slides I had prepared for the talk into the child's history and physical exam, I modeled a pediatric allergy evaluation. I'm confident that few in the audience had experienced this type of clinical teaching before. Later, I learned that from the students' standpoint, this was felt to be an effective presentation. Unfortunately, their faculty didn't appreciate it to the same extent.

How much does a watermelon cost?

In the years after retirement, Diane and I have started going on mission trips to Guatemala with a group of students from a local nursing school. My role is to provide medical coverage for the clinics; Diane provides support in different areas like coordinating the check in process and fitting people for the shoes donated for the clinics.

In eastern Guatemala, growth stunting is a serious public health concern. Our team collects growth data that should allow for more effective nutritional support for these children. Diane also helped with nutrition counseling to combat this problem.

I enjoy teaching nursing students who approach patients from a more holistic perspective than many of the medical students I am more familiar with. Rounds at the Children's Hospital included one-on-one teaching, the type of physician-led training that most nursing students wouldn't have much access to. In rural villages, we performed screening health visits and dispensed anti parasite medications. The nursing students taught villagers the importance of clean water, hand washing, and general hygiene. Many rural families continue to cook indoors over wood burning stoves and suffer greatly from chronic respiratory complaints. Our program provided specially designed cook stoves which were vented to the outside. No more smoke-filled house with every meal. We also brought water filtration systems into their homes to replace their reliance on the often-polluted stream water for drinking and cooking.

As a pediatrician, I was most interested in seeing the children and trying to imagine the lives that awaited them as they grew into adulthood. In one rural village, there were two sisters who expressed their interest in becoming doctors. I let them use my stethoscope to examine their mother and each other. The look of pride on the mother's face was universal; no language barrier here. On other occasions, we conducted clinics adjacent to the city dump where some of the children become victims of human trafficking. Surrounded by dust and decaying garbage and enveloped in a thick cloud of smoke and fog, these people scratch out a living rummaging through other people's garbage. If things go well, they might be able to make a dollar or two per day or find some discarded food to feed their family. It's hard to describe the smell of a setting such as this. Thankfully, one of the nurse practitioners brought along some Vicks VapoRub. A little dab of this under each nostril allowed one to withstand such a smell.

I didn't know any Spanish when we started attending these clinics and tried to ask our drivers about words from time to time. As we were passing a pickup truck loaded down with watermelons, I asked our driver how much one of them would cost in Guatemala. Back at home, these watermelons would certainly have cost five or six dollars or more. He said I should ask the man myself and then gave me instructions on how to do that. "*Cuanto cuesta la sandia*?" This translates to "How much does a watermelon cost?" For the rest of the trip, the standing joke was that the only word I knew in Spanish was translated watermelon. Admittedly, this knowledge was of limited utility in running a medical clinic but at least I knew that I could pick up a watermelon for a dollar.

At one point in His ministry, Jesus criticized the religious leaders who claimed to be serving God even as they ignored the needs of their own families. Like many Bible lessons I had studied, I thought this was a good message for others. Through my work with missions, I found the message was directed toward me as well. Service to others is important, but not at the expense of my own family. I had finally learned to wait patiently for the right time and setting to fulfill my desire to teach. And I wouldn't need to leave my wife behind.

Chapter 17

My First Tattoo, Going from Doctor to Patient

See, I have refined you, but not with silver; I have tested you in the furnace of affliction.

Isaiah 48:10 (NIV)

It is good that I have been afflicted that I might learn your decrees.

Psalm 119:71 (NIV)

A lump in my cheek

Good health is easy to take for granted for someone who has never needed medical care (except for the time I stuck a key in a socket). I took pride in being physically active since running track in high school and playing soccer in college. Later, I enjoyed noncompetitive sports like running, hiking, bicycling, and swimming. My patients were the ones with the serious health problems.

Six months after selling the clinic to the hospital, while still employed full time, I noticed a lump in my cheek. I tried all the usual approaches–denial, hopeful waiting and minimizing the potential problem. That worked until Diane noticed the lump and insisted I get it checked out.

Over lunch at the doctors' lounge, I was speaking with an ENT colleague and shared that I would be seeing him soon for an appointment." He looked at me in a way I had done so many times myself, the times when a diagnosis is made on the spot and didn't waste any time with pleasantries. "I'll see you in my clinic after lunch." (I had just experienced one of the most mysterious aspects of medicine, the blink-of-an-eye diagnosis that doctors make based on experience and intuition.) I rescheduled my afternoon patients and reported to the ENT clinic as instructed.

The surgeon told me what he couldn't say in the doctors' lounge. The lump I had been trying to deny was possibly cancerous. Given its location, a biopsy wouldn't be good enough to make the diagnosis. Surgery would be needed to remove the entire mass and find out what it was. So much for my denial.

I felt like I had returned to medical school for the next few days as I pored over articles and references on facial tumors. It seemed most likely that the tumor was in the parotid gland, one of the main sources of the saliva that makes eating possible. If that were the case, the tumor might be localized to the gland and cured by surgery. Then I started to learn about the other possibilities and they didn't seem so favorable. One way the body protects itself is by stationing lymph nodes to stand guard against local infections. Maybe one of those lymph glands was responsible for my lump.

It's one thing to read about cancer, but no written account could capture the impact of the experience. Within a few days, I would be lying on the bed in the recovery room, groggy and starting to wake up from surgery. Is that the surgeon? What did he say, something about a lump in my parotid gland surrounding the facial nerve? Probably not malignant but can't say for sure. Something didn't look quite right. More tests would be needed. Within a couple of weeks, the final pathology results came in: my lump was due to a cancerous lymph gland located within the parotid gland. How ironic that a physician like myself who specialized in the immune system would now have an immune system tumor.

I didn't realize that my emotional immune system was depleted from the years of independent medical practice and family strain. Though I had sold my practice before learning of the cancer, the stress of working as an employed physician attacked my mental health. Cancer on top of mild depression is a bad combination. Untreated, both could have fatal consequences.

The surgeon had removed the entire tumor, but had it spread? Answering that question required an extensive battery of blood tests, X-rays, and scans to determine the best treatment plan. I had overseen this same sequence of events in my own patients, especially during medical school. TNM: tumor, nodes, mets, that's the way every cancer is evaluated. The testing showed there were no other lymph nodes involved and the tumor had not metastasized or spread anywhere else in my body.

I found it interesting to go through this process as a patient, detached from the reality of my situation, like reading another case report: sixty-five-year-old man with lymphoma confined to the parotid gland...surgery and radiation...good prognosis. Next case...

I blocked out the magnitude of my cancer diagnosis and what it meant for my health, saying that compared to others, I diagnosed myself with "cancer lite." My way of denying the seriousness of my tumor. In truth, everyone knows that cancer is serious. My self-centered "cancer-lite" attitude downplayed the anxieties and fears of those closest to me.

Then reality hit. Maybe mine wasn't the most serious malignancy in the world, but it was still cancer. I began to think of my personal experience with this disease over the course of my career.

Hadn't my dad and sister died from cancer? What about that pain-ridden cancer patient from medical school? Would I suffer like him? How about some of the cancer patients I had cared for and their painful declines and deaths. Images flashed through my mind: the grieving and heartbroken families; the mother who left a husband and their four children behind; the grandmother in hospice, waiting for the end to come; spouses, parents, children, each suffering in their own ways.

The mask

Since my tumor was confined to the left cheek, radiation therapy to this area was recommended. In this form of treatment, beams of high intensity energy are directed into areas of cancer. Ideally, killing any remaining malignant cells before they spread. The radiation beam is incredibly powerful and must be precisely aimed at the right spot or it might miss the tumor and damage healthy tissue. Even being one millimeter off the target could make a difference. It's impossible for anyone to hold still long enough for the treatment, so the patient receives a little help in the form of a fiberglass mesh mask perfectly fitted to the head, neck and upper chest. This is exacting business with no room for error, so the mask is lined up with a dot-sized tattoo placed on the chest. This didn't seem so bad. I even got my first tattoo as a souvenir of the experience and joked that close inspection would reveal a view of the earth from the moon. With the tattoo and mask, the reality of my diagnosis and the radiation treatment hit.

So much of my life had been spent in an effort to maintain control over my circumstances, but now I was completely under the control of someone else. A radiation treatment session starts with getting positioned on the cold, hard radiation treatment table surrounded by a team of nurses and technicians. Once they were satisfied with my positioning, they retrieved my personal mask from a rack of masks on the side of the room. I watched them line up the mask with my chest tattoo , the fiberglass pressing against my face. So far, not too bad, until the nurse started securing the mask to the treatment table with a set of bolts, like lug nuts holding a tire in place. One by one, the bolts are screwed down, tighter and tighter, until no movement is possible. That's when the problems started. The mask squeezed my Adam's apple. Breathing became more difficult and I could no longer swallow. Thoughts of choking to death raced through my mind. I was sure that had never happened there before, but…

Finally, completely affixed to the table, like some specimen from high school biology lab, it was time for the treatment to begin. The technicians retreated to the safety of the control room, leaving me all alone, at the mercy of the invisible, undetectable radiation beam whose sole purpose was to kill any cells directly in its path. The only sensations were occasional clicking sounds, some movement of the machine, and flashing lights, my own personal laser show.

Each day for the next three weeks I reported to the radiation therapy unit for my treatment. After a few pleasantries, I braced myself for the mask with not very helpful self-talk like, "It wouldn't take much for this mask to choke me altogether. What if they forgot about me and weren't there to rescue me if I got into trouble? What if the machine just went wild, like I was in some late-night science fiction movie?" All of this went through my head as I lay bolted to the table straining for each breath.

I have some difficulty with claustrophobia anyway so I generally avoid tight spaces. I couldn't avoid the mask but I could avoid the negative thinking. The radiation therapy required a great deal of positive self-talk to get through the treatment process. But these radiation treatments were necessary if I wanted to make sure my cancer was completely treated. My head reminded me that breathing difficulties can come from anxiety. "Just relax; you'll get through this." How many times had I given that advice to my patients? Now I was one of them.

I thought back to earlier times when I had breathing difficulties when swimming in a triathlon or across a lake. In both cases my mind would sabotage my efforts with thoughts like, "This water is really deep, and it doesn't matter if you've trained for the swim. You could drown and nobody would know it. Maybe you should wear a depth finder in case you go down."

The impact of radiation therapy extended beyond killing any cancer cells that might have remained. Any treatment strong enough to kill cancer cells has the potential to cause side effects as well. Some people suffer damage to the skin or underlying tissues; my side effects were different. I don't think there are any cells in the body responsible for a person having a sense of pride, but if there are, mine withered under that radiation beam.

I had spent much of my life proudly self-reliant and unsure of the reliability of others. Now I found myself totally at the mercy of the radiation therapist and his staff and absolutely had to trust them.

While emotionally difficult, the radiation therapy experience was a spiritually engaging time. For the first time, I confronted my own mortality. I had dedicated my life to promoting the health of others. Now it was my turn to receive care. At home, I devoted extra attention to looking for Bible verses that might relate to my situation, my family, and my purpose in life.

When the time came for a radiation treatment, I would enter the treatment room reviewing my trusty scripture index card. As the session progressed, I'd refer back to that card or other Bible verses I'd previously memorized. I would think of Scripture passages that I had been teaching to others such as a passage from the Psalms which tells us we can call out to God who fulfills His purpose for us. But what was His purpose for me now? Sometimes, praise and worship music would come to mind. Trusting God and employing these spiritual practices helped me successfully complete the radiation treatments. More than that, they redirected my thinking.

Once I had recovered from the surgery and radiation therapy, I returned to work, even though I had been given the option of early retirement, no questions asked. Working one more year was part of the practice sale agreement. I wanted to honor my contract and heed my mother's advice from many years earlier, "Once a job is first begun, never leave it 'til it's done..." Or was refusing to retire actually just another way of denying my cancer?

Cancer makes another house call

It's nice to think that the cancer patient could simply move on after treatment through prayer, positive thinking, or mindfulness, but is that possible? Every shower provides a fresh opportunity to find something unexpected. I occasionally perform lymph node exams even without thinking about it. Shaving becomes an occasion to check for any new lumps in my cheek.

As I neared the end of the observation period for the lymphoma treatment, I noticed a small sore on my left ear in the area of the radiation treatment. Denial didn't make it go away this time either so I eventually consulted my doctor. A biopsy showed the sore was skin cancer. More tests. Another surgery, then more follow-up visits to ensure that there was no recurrence. A sigh of relief–two cancers successfully treated over a period of five years. I was officially in the clear, but a nagging concern about some suspicious prostate findings meant it was time to make acquaintances with a urologist who suggested a biopsy be obtained.

The results came in an unexpected way. Diane and I had just finished our third mission trip to Guatemala with the nursing students and were taking a few days of vacation in the scenic historic capital city of Antigua. Sitting in a coffee shop enjoying a latte, I took an incoming call. It was my urologist who called to tell me that the biopsy showed I had low-grade prostate cancer. I understood this to be a common problem for many men and not much to be cause for concern and commented to that effect. "It may be low grade, but you still have cancer. You're going to need more tests and possible treatment." Reality once again prevailed over my dismissive thinking. My dad had died from this disease as did my medical school patient with the severe bone pain. No more joking about "cancer lite."

In medical school we questioned how a physician could truly understand the patient's experience with a condition having never actually experienced it themselves. The doctor may try to empathize with the patient but is always bound to come up short. I found I could now speak about cancer with others from personal experience. My cancer journey has made it possible to talk to them in ways not previously possible. I am better equipped to advise family members and to teach valuable lessons to medical students as well. I've also become familiar with the Sting Cancer movement, a place to meet cancer patients and survivors surrounded by family, friends, all supporting each other. And now I will always be one of them.

A physician doesn't generally have the luxury of dealing with only one thing at a time given the frequent interruptions, emergencies, and other demands for their attention inherent in a medical setting. Throughout my career, I had prided myself in being able to partition my thinking to keep from getting too emotionally involved with my patients' problems. This ability to compartmentalize my thinking may have kept the problems of life from interfering with my medical practice. The downside of boxing up emotions is that the box might never be examined.

When first diagnosed with cancer, I planned to follow this same detached approach. Cancer wasn't going to conquer me. I might slow down a bit for a while, but I wasn't going to take extra time off like others did. I would get back to work as though nothing had happened, except that I had a little less energy than before. In retrospect, this prideful attitude was a big mistake. I needed time to heal physically and emotionally. Maybe I was reliving my reaction to receiving that penicillin shot in the dining room when I tried to get out of going to school. "Good, we've caught it in time. Now you can get back to school."

A new perspective

On a positive note, my cancer experience has encouraged me to maintain good health through exercise with varying degrees of success. I enjoy running and walking and have run several marathons and other races. I was training for a half marathon when I discovered the lump in my cheek. Most people newly diagnosed with a life-threatening illness wouldn't spend a Sunday morning in the spring running 13.1 miles with thousands of their closest friends. I saw the race as a great challenge that would motivate me in my recovery.

Though I had run many road races before, surgery and radiation had weakened me more than I realized. I could now barely walk around the block, much less run any distance, especially in the winter. Getting outside was going to be a challenge. For the next couple of months, Diane would walk with me around the block, holding my arm to keep me from falling until I could walk and eventually run on my own. She patiently helped me regain my strength and cheered me on when I completed the half marathon that spring.

For each of the next four springs, I ran the half marathon race but with a new outlook. No more competing for a personal best time for me. No more trying to get ahead of some other runners and beat them to the finish line. Instead, I made special note of the many participants who had t-shirts dedicated to loved ones suffering from cancer or some other health problem. Sometimes I ran alongside them and asked about their stories. Every runner is in the race for a reason. Something motivated them and I wanted to find out what that was. Over the almost 3 hours it took to complete the race, I met several other runners who had been treated for cancer. Though they were complete strangers, we shared a common bond.

After being diagnosed with cancer three different times, I no longer see other people with chronic health problems in the same way. They each have stories of hopes and fears, triumphs and setbacks, and are hopefully surrounded by supportive loved ones. It's all about how we see things, and my perspective had changed. With my recent introduction to mindfulness, I began to see the value of looking at each day in the present, not ruminating about the past or worrying about the future. Getting sick didn't stop me from working, but it certainly contributed to my later decision to retire altogether. If work-related stress didn't cause my cancer, it wasn't helping my immune system's effort to recover. I had to make changes in my lifestyle and work.

Chapter 18

I'm Indispensable, Right?

Moses was 120 years old when he died, yet his eyesight was clear and he was as strong as ever.

Deuteronomy 34:7 (NLT)

With the diagnosis of cancer, came the realization that I wouldn't be able to work indefinitely, nor would I even want to. I had been striving all my life to gain the acceptance and approval of others. While successful in many ways, this misguided quest kept me from taking the time needed to recover from surgery and radiation. Retirement started looking more attractive. All along, retirement was going to be solely under my control, on my own terms, and at my own time. But the world has a habit of getting in the way of carefully thought-out plans.

Two doctors talking

There's the story of the two older doctors discussing their plans with the office staff. Both see themselves as indispensable. The first doctor announces their pending retirement and receives comments like, "Really, so soon? How can you consider leaving us and your patients? We need you to continue." The second doctor gets a different response. Outwardly, the staff talks in glowing terms about the doctor's career of service but inwardly, it's a different matter: "Finally! We thought the day would never come. How soon can we have the retirement party? What kind of cake would you like?"

I was determined to be that first doctor, the one who still provided unrivaled medical care up to the last day of practice. Doctors who continued to practice beyond their time were like aging athletes hanging on for one more season of glory, their identities wrapped up in career and performance. My identity was bound up in being a doctor. Without patients to care for, who or what am I?

As chairman of the hospital's physician health committee, I knew all about the concept of physician burnout. This was a definite problem for many other physicians but certainly not for me. At least, that's what I thought. My practice style emphasized making personal connections with patients, a high maintenance approach that required a lot of emotional energy. I was wearing myself down, and something clearly wasn't right in my thinking and self-talk like in dialogues like this:

Speaking to myself: "Sometimes, I wonder how much good I've actually done for my patients."

Listening to others: "Look at all the people you're helping around here."

Response to myself: "I suppose that's true, but look at all the ones that haven't gotten better. Maybe they would be better off under the care of someone else."

It's often said that people don't often leave their job; they leave their managers. Having sold my practice to the hospital, I no longer had final say on how the office would be staffed or operated. When I stated to the manager that the clinic environment seemed hostile, I was probably voicing my final plea for help. Rather than opening up a needed conversation, my comments were dismissed. Since childhood, I had backed away from directly expressing my deepest feelings to others. That non-confrontational style took away my final chance to salvage my job.

Nor did the hospital administration seem to care either about my growing dissatisfaction at work. Upon announcing my retirement plans, I was completely unprepared to find that they didn't want to keep me on staff. Like that over-the-hill athlete, I was to be replaced with a young recruit. All my life, I had been able to work my way out of problems by studying them and then making needed changes in my approach. This time, the problems were too great and the obstacles too immovable for me to prevail. All that was left for me was to decide what kind of cake I wanted.

A different kind of mask

I was now trapped in a negative feedback loop en route to hopelessness and isolation. In my mind, physicians weren't supposed to show weakness or share personal problems, even when the emotions are raw and the disappointments are great. My years of self-protective silence kept me from sharing my deepest feelings with anyone except my wife, and even she only heard some of my inner dialogue. Years earlier, I had hinted at some of this negative inner thinking during a visit with my personal physician. Seeing the alarmed look on his face, I quickly downplayed the comment about my mood and changed the subject, fearful he might refer me for counseling. Easier to change the subject to diet, exercise, and cholesterol. Better to keep my emotions to myself. Looking back, my radiation therapy mask had been replaced by a mask of my own construction, self-inflicted but equally suffocating.

Faced with a work situation I couldn't resolve and concerns about my health, I finally accepted that it was time to change. The best thing I could do was to honor my contract and then move on in life. After all, "Once a job is first begun, never leave it 'til it's done..."

Chapter 19

So Where Does That Leave Me in Retirement?

The righteous flourish like the palm tree and grow like a cedar in Lebanon. They are planted in the house of the LORD; they flourish in the courts of our God. They still bear fruit in old age; they are ever full of sap and green, to declare that the LORD is upright.

Psalm 92:12–15a (ESV)

Retire (verb)

To withdraw from one's position or occupation; conclude one's working or professional career

To withdraw from action or danger: Retreat

To go to bed

To cause to retire from one's position occupation

To put out (as in a batter in baseball)

Source: Merriam-Webster Dictionary

What does it mean to retire? Originally referring to a turning back to safety, the word "retire" later took on additional meanings such as withdrawing troops from battle or leaving an occupation, especially due to age or to collect Social Security. In my thinking, retirement was going to be my choice and on my terms. It never crossed my mind that "retire" can also be something done *to* a person against their will, like in baseball, where to be retired means to be put out. For me retirement was more a matter of finding that hospital management was not interested in offering a part-time contract.

As long as I was busy raising a family and seeing patients, I was able to avoid challenging the story I had enshrined in my set way of thinking–I was abandoned by my dad when he left home and moved away. Within a few years of his leaving, I would become the oldest one of the kids remaining at home, and I was responsible for helping my mother and younger siblings while being self-reliant in directing my own life. I believed I was valued and accepted most for what I could successfully accomplish.

For years, this narrative played over and over in my head and guided my thinking. How many times did I replay that scene in Dad's office when he told us once and for all that he was leaving? How many times did I make choices based on my conviction that success in life was based on doing good things so I could gain the approval of others? This was the script of my life and I followed it faithfully until I couldn't any longer.

There didn't seem to be any way out of this continuous memory loop until I started examining my story more critically. In the process, I discovered that writing my story has a power of its own. As a physician, I composed accurate patient care notes to record the medical encounters. Writing my own story isn't just a matter of recording the past; it has also given me greater peace in the present and helped me anticipate a brighter future. Writing became my way of coming to grips with my life's story, and rewriting its script from one of painful abandonment and loss to a hopeful one of trust and acceptance.

Discovering these new insights required traveling far back into childhood to unearth and examine long-buried memories and find answers to the questions that have been with me much of my life. I needed to take a hard look at how birth order, parental alcoholism, and divorce became the three interwoven strands defining my life. I reflected on how these three realities came together to shape me, each contributing something to my life, much as a mix of spices interact with each other to create a distinct aroma and flavor.

Family life

I will repay you for the years the locusts have eaten.

Joel 2:25 (ESV)

Much of my life had been about reaching the destination, continually looking forward to whatever was coming next, like the tourist too obsessed with the guidebook to enjoy the scenery. Delayed gratification formed the foundation of medical training. As we walked through neighborhoods while in medical school, Diane and I used to admire the brick houses with their furnishings and cars. We were certain that leaving our one-bedroom apartment and attaining all of this would make us happy. Now we have our own cars and a well-furnished house and realize these things aren't the answer. Throughout the years in school, I looked forward to getting out of the classroom and into the workplace. Now that I've been on the job for over 40 years, I just think about getting back to school.

Before we started our family, it seemed that having children would fulfill our dreams. Soon we were outnumbered by children and we began looking for a respite from the day-to-day pressures of parenting. Much later, we looked forward to launching our kids, but now we look for ways to repopulate our empty nest with our grandchildren. For many people, retirement is the great sustaining dream throughout their working careers. But that wasn't the case for me. Retirement was never my final destination. I saw it as a time to pursue life beyond the workplace. I didn't anticipate that retirement would cause me to face the tough questions of life and come to grips with who I was.

Earlier in life, my focus had been on compensating for childhood losses by striving for success through hard work. But my zeal to overcome these shortcomings often caused new problems for me and my family. Aristotle said we become what we repeatedly do. In keeping busy all the time with work and my own interests, I showed those things were my highest priorities. But that wasn't the kind of person I wanted to be.

My identity had been based on my work and accomplishments, a sort of perpetual family dinner with Dad at the head of the table with up to a dozen children competing for his attention. Back then, I came armed with report cards, awards, newspaper articles, and scholarships to show my work. What would I have to show for myself now?

I was beginning to see life through a different set of eyes. Before my own health problems surfaced, Diane and I started spending more time with her mother whose health was starting to decline. This usually involved Mary Lou coming to our home for a day or two. One day, we asked her when she wanted a ride back to her apartment. "Never," she replied. She lived in our home from that point on, first in an upstairs bedroom and eventually in a hospital bed in our family room.

I loved being in a position to serve the woman who had done so much to keep Diane and me together when we were first dating. When the time came that she could no longer get out of bed without assistance, we had to find a way for her to get our attention. After an intercom and doorbell proved to be too noisy, we settled on a whistle. One day, Mary Lou had some visitors and we heard the whistle calling us. We rushed into the family room afraid of what problem might have arisen. But there was our smiling patient sitting up in bed with the whistle in hand. "I just wanted to show my friends that all I had to do was blow the whistle and you would come running." Before long, hospice got involved, preparing us all for what was to come. Mary Lou passed away in our family room a few months later, surrounded by her loving family.

While Mary Lou was in her final months, another tragedy struck our family. This was the day my son Tony and his wife Anna were going to close on the purchase of their new home. The moving truck was being loaded and they were busy with the countless details involved with moving when tragedy struck. While sitting in his infant seat, their 7-week-old baby Linus stopped breathing. Just like that. One moment alive and well, the next another victim of SIDS. One moment, the growing family is happily looking forward to their new home; the next, they are overcome with grief.

I was working in the clinic when the panic-stricken call came to the office. Something about Linus and paramedics and get home right away. I left the clinic in the middle of a patient visit and rushed home to pick up Diane and Mary Lou. When we arrived at the home where Tony and Anna were staying, the house was crowded with sobbing family, police officers, EMTs and the coroner. Resuscitation efforts were unsuccessful. Linus was taken to the morgue where an autopsy confirmed that he had died of SIDS.

My mind went back to the time when Linus was several weeks old. His mom called me one evening with concerns about the way he was nursing. I examined him in our living room and couldn't find anything wrong. The next day, I called their pediatrician to discuss their concerns and the normal exam just to be safe. In the aftermath of his death, I reviewed the situation and questioned whether I had overlooked something when I had examined Linus. Could the death of our grandson have been prevented? I don't believe so, but with SIDS, there are many more questions than answers.

We never really talked as a family about how SIDS had robbed us all of that precious baby boy. We never shared our bewilderment that some mysterious condition could claim the life of a healthy-appearing baby at any time of the day or night. We never reassured each other that nothing could have been done to prevent this tragedy. No, we buried our questions and emotions along with that tiny white flower-covered casket. The whole family went back to their lives, grieving privately, as if life would somehow return to normal. But it never did.

Teacher–Going from clinic to classroom

God gave some to be…pastors and teachers

Ephesians 4:11 (ESV)

Now teach these truths to other trustworthy people who will be able to pass them on to others.

2 Timothy 2:2 (NLT)

During high school, my career dilemma involved choosing between being a doctor or a teacher. It never occurred to me at the time that I could be both. (In Latin class, I had learned that the word doctor actually comes from the Latin word *docere* "*to teach*.") Teaching has always interested me, and I embraced every opportunity. In college, that meant demonstrating science experiments in community settings. Medical school was the time to prepare a lecture and deliver it to my class. The professor had an air of self importance that prompted me to have myself paged during my presentation. I interrupted the talk to write the urgent message on the chalkboard: Remember the eggs, milk and bread. In residency, came recognition for my bedside teaching on the wards. During the allergy training, the fellows taught the medical students and residents rotating through the clinic. In clinical practice, the staff were always in need of training, and patient care visits typically involved teaching the patient and family as well. Altogether, I had received quite a bit of encouragement to be a teacher throughout my educational journey, but I lacked the confidence to teach at a medical school until late in my career.

That changed with the startup of the Medical College of Wisconsin (MCW) campus in Green Bay. This was my first contact with the school my father and brother had attended at its main campus in Milwaukee. Joining their faculty enabled me to follow in my father's footsteps in another way. I became involved on the ground floor, when courses were being prepared from scratch, just as I had done in college. My role involved developing and teaching courses for medical students at the beginning stages of their careers. This made it possible for me to emphasize the importance of treating each patient as an individual, just as I had tried to do in my own practice. In seeing patients on my own, I had cared for thousands of individuals. Taken together, our small class of twenty-five students might care for several million patients over their collective careers, reflecting the exponential impact of a single teacher.

My main problem in this new role was balancing two different jobs. There was so much new information to learn if I were to be an effective teacher, but I was still trying to care for patients in the clinic. I tried reading books on medical education and applying them to my teaching. This helped me learn education theory, but I still had to decide how these insights should be put into practice. How does one try new approaches and tailor their instruction to the everchanging capabilities of the students without overwhelming them in the process?

Teaching the course on professional development yielded unanticipated benefits. Our session on care of persons with disabilities gave Sam the opportunity to speak to the class about his personal experience of living with quadriplegia. The students received firsthand reports of what it was like to be paralyzed, blind, or deaf from Sam and the other speakers. They learned that disabled persons can't take anything for granted, even something as simple as getting out of bed. And the medical students weren't the only ones to benefit from this session. Sam and the other speakers also found that sharing their stories helped them find purpose and meaning in their own challenges.

The session on geriatrics introduced me to people in the community who serve older adults. For the class, I was also able to recruit Maryl Hitchcock, a former patient of mine, to speak to the students. Maryl informed them that she was 95½ years old (and don't forget the ½) and described her life as a wife, mother, and former teacher. The experience was so good for her that Maryl invited the class out for dinner to continue the discussion. Through working together at school, Maryl and I have developed a friendship that extends far beyond the classroom.

In embracing my role as a medical educator, I had finally overcome the lack of confidence that had held me back for so many years. My practice days were coming to an end, but my dream of teaching was coming true and with it came a chance to develop new skills and serve in new ways. Whatever I might bring to our students came from the lessons learned through years of clinical practice.

Volunteer

And let us not grow weary of doing good, for in due season we will reap, if we do not give up.

Galatians 6:9 (ESV)

"Whatever you did for one of the least of these brothers and sisters of mine, you did for me."

Matthew 25: 40 (NIV)

After my retirement, I started getting involved with local volunteer work and service. Our daughter Rachel had accepted a position at the New Community Shelter where they provided meals and housing for the homeless and the working poor. Diane and I took a tour of the shelter and for the first time, came to appreciate the tremendous needs of the homeless population. I began to volunteer at the evening meals a couple of times per month. My job was to serve milk, coffee, and juice while keeping the beverage station as clean and presentable as possible. This was my first direct contact with homeless persons where I could meet them face to face, and get to know them as people.

One day, I was getting ready to help serve a lunch meal when the tornado sirens warned us to take shelter. Everyone, residents, guests, and volunteers headed into a stairwell to ride out the storm. This became my opportunity to talk to them one on one, the same diners I'd been serving at my beverage station. They told of their families, and of their broken homes, broken careers, broken dreams. Our relationship no longer revolved around a cup of coffee or glass of milk. This experience transformed my thinking about the homeless and prompted me to write an essay about our conversations. Writing about the experience taught me much about myself. I had always seen myself as quite different from the homeless and working poor. But was I really all that different? Didn't we all share the same hopes and dreams for ourselves and our families? Having the writing published gave me a new forum to speak out for the needs of others.

During another dinner at the shelter, an older gentleman wearing a cowboy hat and Western style jacket carefully added milk and sugar to his cup of coffee. Splash! Coffee, milk and sugar spilled all over my spotless beverage station. Who would have guessed that a previous diner had unscrewed the cover to the sugar dispenser? "So sorry," said the guest in halting English. "It was an accident," I reassured him. "We'll just call your drink, *Mucho azúcar con poco café.*" (A lot of sugar with a little coffee). He smiled at my attempted Spanish and thanked me. A few weeks later, we met again. As he came to get his coffee, I greeted him and told him we could call him, "*Señor Mucho azúcar con poco café.*" He smiled at the recognition and each mealtime we talked, he told me a little more about himself, his journey from the Dominican Republic to Green Bay and his love of music, his dream of finding a place of his own. All these discoveries made possible from spilling a little sugar.

Following our parents' example, my siblings and I have continued to serve, each one applying some special gift or ability for the benefit of others. Some examples: Mary Barbara, the prison nurse, Kathy, teaching English as a Second Language; Mark, the retired judge serving on the board of directors for school and community groups; Joe, providing for a family member with special needs; Johnny, the musician producing a music CD to raise funds for soup kitchens; Margaret, the family historian serving nieces and nephews at times of need; Jane, who volunteers to teach at her grandchildren's school; Nancy, singing at church; Amy, bringing meals to shut-ins; Lora, the visiting nurse; Luke, the doctor, serving at summer camps; and Lucy, reading the Scriptures at church. (One of my siblings pointed out that each of us has chosen a career that emphasized control of circumstances in some way or other. Was this our way of achieving the sense of control we had missed out on earlier in life?) Several years ago, the role of our family in the community was recognized. Together, we received a Families of Distinction Award sponsored by the YWCA, a testimony to the values instilled in us by our parents.

Each member of my own family has also begun serving in our community using their own gifts and talents. Diane volunteers with the local Master Gardener Program. Rachel, Emily, and Peter have worked in community service-related programs and Tony, has played on the worship team at church. Each of our children also serve as Sam's caregivers. Sam has used his business experience to organize fundraisers that support social-justice-related concerns. He now shares his life story with community groups. Our grandchildren are now continuing this legacy of service. Madeline, our teenage granddaughter, is serving with a peer mediation program at her high school. As a first grader, our grandson Elijah collected coffee mugs for the homeless shelter. Four generations of service.

Writer

Thus says the Lord, the God of Israel, "Write in a book all the words that I have spoken to you."

Jeremiah 30:2 (ESV)

I don't know that I would ever have completely broken free of the script that was directing my life if it hadn't been for writing. As I began to record my life experiences, I found it necessary to discuss them with my siblings. In part, this was my effort to check the accuracy of my memories, but at a deeper level, it also gave me a chance to hear their stories. We talk freely now of memories submerged in the silence of a home where sharing thoughts and feelings was discouraged.

Our shared experiences affected each of us in different ways, in part because we each sat at a different place at the table when Dad came to town. We were at different ages and stages of development when major life events dominated our family's life. Remarkable how members of a family can come from the same background yet still have very different experiences.

Through my teaching at the medical school, I introduced reflective writing to my medical students in our course on professional development. Medical literature suggests that this type of writing helps students develop empathic thinking. As it became clear that our students were benefiting in this way from their writing, reflective writing became a required part of their training.

So, what would prompt a retired doctor to take up yet another encore career, this time as a writer? I think there's always been a writer in me, dormant in expression but always present, a seed waiting for the right conditions to germinate. In high school, we learned about diagramming sentences, an orderly arrangement of all the nouns, verbs, clauses, and modifiers, each in its place. Perfect for someone who likes order. I enjoyed writing in college and recall writing an essay about the swamp and river near my boyhood home. Was that my first effort at a memoir? When I wrote a paper about the movie *Gone with the Wind*, two of my sisters loved the book and my paper so much they paid to use it to meet the demands of their own coursework. Does this make me a professional writer?

Writing poetry was interesting, although I never considered it one of my strong points. Diane indulged me in this and received many poems and little notes to celebrate birthdays and anniversaries. Sometimes she would get a short poem with her morning coffee or with some flowers, usually based on *Roses are red…* I still have some of these early attempts at poetry in our family scrapbook and will spare the reader the pain of bringing them forth.

Other poetic efforts were a little more expressive, as with this note accompanying a gift of flowers:

The Cyclamen
May the freshness, beauty and new life of this cyclamen
Remind us that true love is
Always budding with new possibilities

Through our children, I became interested in haiku and tried my hand at that as well:

God's hand
Flowers bloom afresh
Squirrels frolic playfully
God's hand in nature

A Learning in Retirement program introduced me to the concept of using writing as a means of overcoming personal trauma. I already knew that I often felt better after getting my thoughts down on paper but didn't know there was research that confirmed this. In their book *Expressive Writing, Words That Heal* James Pennebaker and John Evans demonstrated that writing in a structured way helped people recover from some of the trials and traumas of life. With this new understanding, I started to share this technique with my children and others. We've had trouble talking about the traumas our family has experienced. With time, our shared writing may help us know each other better and experience healing as a family.

The program also showed how poetry and creative writing helped express emotions too hard to talk about directly. Reflecting on the loss of our grandson:

Grief
Grief
Stored away
In the closet
Deal with it later
Time is now
Spring cleaning
Acceptance

Only in the writing of this memoir did I finally put my feelings into the following words on the occasion of what would have been Linus' eighth birthday:

No Cake
no cake
party or presents
no games
balloons or face painting
no laughter
only silence
across the street
from the school he never saw
one less child on the playground

I find it's often helpful to express information I'm learning in different ways. This often helps me see new relationships not readily apparent from listening to a talk or reading an article. A speaker at a nearby college was presenting data on the impact of technology on our society's growing problem with personal relationships. In response to the talk, I composed the following:

Unanswered
Wordless, relationship in peril
Once intimate, now grown sterile
Bids unanswered, hopes unseen
Attention blocked, the ever-present screen
Yet each bid bears fresh potential
And response essential, consequential
Jagged, tough, seeming a stone
The hurt one pleads, "Put down that phone."

Regular journaling never came easy to me as evidenced by a shelf full of partly used journals, notebooks, and legal pads each with only a few pages of notes. With more time available in retirement, I now write daily journal entries and find this to be a good way to clarify my thoughts and address my concerns about daily life. Sometimes, these reflections become the basis for an extended reflection, my personal "Thought for the Day" and possible material for another book.

I've come to see that all my life experiences, from early family life to having a family of my own, the years of education and medical practice have together prepared me to write. I'm no longer afraid to identify myself as a writer and author or to encourage my family to write a collective memoir. Our family's story needs to be told to others.

It's been said that writers should wait to tell their story until they've recovered from their traumas. I can see the value of waiting until the emotions have tempered with time and reflection. However, for me, the act of writing has changed my understanding of life's events. Taking the time to carefully write out my story has helped me find and accept myself and my family. In doing so, I came to understand that all along, my life has been a living play, with each scene carefully arranged to fashion me into the person I've become.

In a sense, I am an actor, freely choosing how to express myself. God is the director who has a part in arranging the scenes.

Epilogue

Donuts and Strawberry Jam

For we are God's handiwork created in Christ Jesus to do good works which he has prepared in advance for us to do.

Ephesians 2:10 (ESV)

My best memory is the time I read in bed with my dad. He taught me many lessons and inspired me to serve others, from our home town to the mission field. In writing about our relationship, I came to understand how much we had in common.

Dad's final bed rests on a hillside in the Catholic Cemetery across the street from his great grandchildren's elementary school, where his daughter served as principal. Dad is flanked on his right by his beloved MaryAnn; on the left, lies my own infant grandson, Linus. Nearby, several of his children have secured their own spots for future use. Once again, Dad has assumed his proud position as patriarch, surrounded by loved ones.

It has been a long time coming, but my quest to rewrite the script has been rewarded with a deeper appreciation for my family, starting with my parents and siblings. I've been able to recognize the strengths and shortcomings of each person in my own family. Diane and I share our family traditions with our grandchildren such as baking, playing games, doing puzzles, and picking strawberries for making homemade jam.

In my childhood, feeling sick would have been dealt with through an injection, and I would be headed off to school. When our grandchildren aren't feeling well and can't go to school, they come to our house for the day for games (and maybe a little rest.) Elijah and I have started the "Early Risers" club where we read together, much like I had done with my dad. We have even talked about writing a children's story together. Our granddaughter Frannie works in the arts and crafts center in our dining room.We are active contributors to the lives of our grandchildren in ways I never experienced as a child, although I must admit, my strawberry jam is no match for my grandma's sugar donuts!

Acknowledgements

The way of a fool is right in his own eyes, but a wise man listens to advice.

Proverbs 12:15 (ESV)

Writing a book about one's life story doesn't just happen without the encouragement and support of many others, especially family. My wife Diane has graciously encouraged me through all the steps of writing. I am so thankful for her loving support. My children have also been very supportive of this effort, though it opens up some painful memories. Perhaps they will write their own story of our family's response to tragedy. My siblings, especially Nancy Schultz and Amy Warpinski patiently reviewed my writing and helped me fill in the gaps in my family background. Margaret DeBruine helped with the photos.

My friend Sterling Swan has been a source of support for many years. When his wife Karen became critically ill with a brain tumor, Sterling became her 24/7 caregiver until the end of her life. His intimate account of his caregiver experience, *Woman on the Bed*, motivated me to write my own story.

Our friends Jack and Kathy Wagoner patiently challenged my thinking about faith as I came to develop a deep relationship with God. They are now helping me revise this account of my life story.

Pastor Paul Garrison introduced me to Biblical Greek and taught me to use that knowledge to strengthen my Bible teaching.

My trusted friend and business consultant Jeff Bramschreiber guided me through my career in practice and joined me on the mission field

Professionally, I owe my involvement in the new medical school to Morgan Rabatine Nagel and Dean Matthew Hunsaker. I have had the great privilege of being part of the inaugural Kinetic3 program of the Kern Institute at the Medical College of Wisconsin through the encouragement of Dr. Kristina Kaljo. The Kern Institute emphasizes the importance of physicians developing the qualities of Caring, Character, and Competence in their professional lives. I appreciate the confidence shown in me by MCW physicians Bruce Campbell and Linda Meurer who encouraged my growth as a medical educator and writer. Just as in practicing clinical medicine, no teacher could function without the contributions of the many staff members including Dana Daggs, Sousie Lee, and Tammy Hosch. I am thankful for their encouragement and support.

Many accomplished writers, artists, and scientists are surrounded by other men and women of stature. These are the people who challenged each other's thinking to bring out the best in their lives. Since my life has been lived in more modest circumstances, I have drawn on the wisdom of others through the many books I've read over the years. Some of these have had an outstanding effect on my life. My thinking certainly wouldn't be the same without them.

Chief among these would be the Bible, which I have been reading through each year for about the last twenty-five years, three or four chapters per day. It's amazing how much God's Word has to say about my daily life and even about circumstances that don't appear to be directly related to the Scriptures. In this regard, I'm thankful for the Bible study where I learned the value of the index card. With that simple tool, I have been able to share the Bible with anyone who expressed interest. People are hungry for the truth even if they are not necessarily interested in the Christian perspective.

Some mentors come in the form of teachers and guides. Others come through the literature and stories we encounter. An Emily Dickenson poem learned in high school English class would shape a lifetime of thinking about the importance of the inner thought life.

To make a prairie
To make a prairie it takes a clover and one bee
one clover and a bee
and reverie
and reverie alone will do
if bees are few

Mars Hill Audio Journals and their discussion of the interaction of culture and Christian thinking have been regular companions for over thirty years.

The writings of Dr. John Patrick have helped shape my thinking about matters of Christian and the cultural assumptions that underlie our society's current thinking.

The Great Courses have been another of my regular companions over the years. I love learning new things from great teachers and especially appreciate the ones who have helped me become a better teacher myself. The list of relevant great courses is lengthy but would have to include those by Professors Michael Roberto and J. Rufus Fears, as well as series on storytelling, writing, mindfulness, music, cognitive neuroscience, and psychology.

My editors Joanne Nelson and Kim Suhr patiently helped me learn how to tell my story.

I'm thankful for my patients who have enriched my life in ways I could never have imagined. They have helped me appreciate the human condition and the complexity of the human body. Serving them has been my great motivator. It has been a great privilege to be a member of their personal care team and now to teach the lessons they taught me to their future physicians. I could never have cared for them without devoted staff, including Michelle Lampereur and my son Tony Warpinski.

Most of all, I want to acknowledge God who has given me all these experiences of life and who sustains me each day. Scripture tells us that it's God who chooses when and where each person will be born. I'm continually thankful that He has chosen this time and place for me. I pray that this account of my life will bring glory to Him.

About The Author

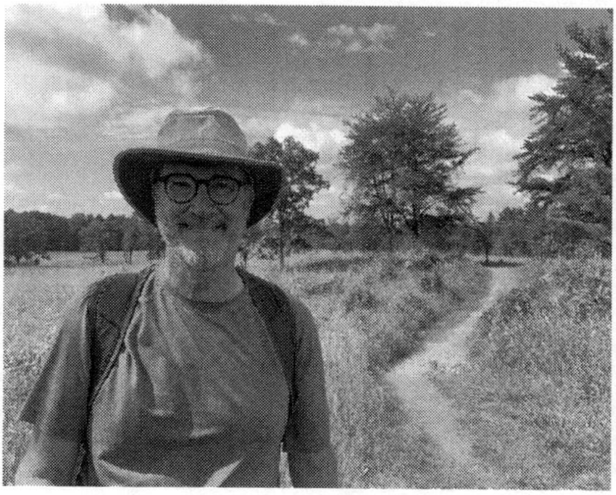

Dr James Warpinski is a retired physician turned writer and medical educator. His essays in medical and lay publications share his experiences as a volunteer at a homeless shelter and as a three-time cancer survivor. Child number six of fourteen in a family fractured by the death of a child leading to alcoholism and eventual parental divorce, he reflects on his lifetime efforts to overcome early life abandonment, workplace betrayal and family tragedy. His memoir, *Rewriting the Script*, depicts the struggles of a doctor trying to balance family and professional life in a culture that demands full allegiance from its healers.

Dr. James Warpinski now teaches medical students about professional development, drawing on his lifetime of experience with the good and bad in American medicine. He and his wife Diane live in Green Bay WI and enjoy gardening, reading, cooking, and sharing life with their five grown children and three grandchildren. They have served on short-term medical missions and are currently writing an account of their experience hiking Wisconsin's National Scenic Ice Age Trail.

Reach the author at: www.jameswarpinskimd.com where he shares his perspectives on life, medicine, and faith.

Can You Help?

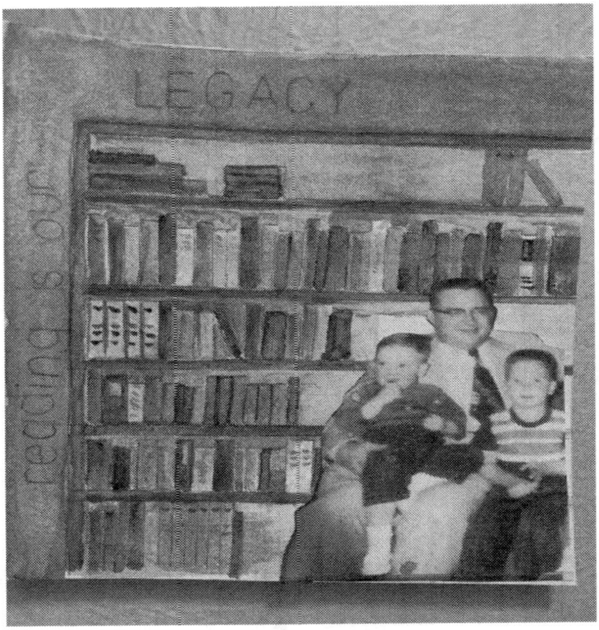

With Dad and my older brother Joe

Thank You For Reading My Book!

I really appreciate all of your feedback, and I love hearing what you have to say.

I need your input to make the next version of this book and my future books better.

Please leave me an honest review on Amazon letting me know what you thought of the book.

Thanks so much!

Dr. James Warpinski

Made in the USA
Monee, IL
10 December 2023

47842209R00159